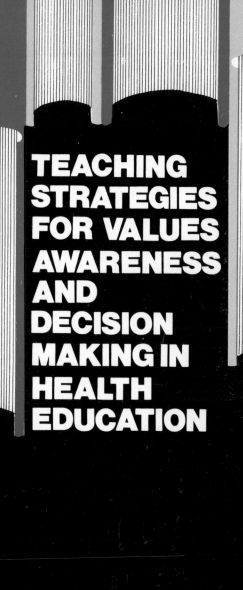

TEACHING
STRATEGIES
FOR VALUES
AWARENESS
AND
DECISION
MAKING IN
HEALTH
EDUCATION

Gus T. Dalis and Ben B. Strasser

TEACHING STRATEGIES FOR VALUES AWARENESS AND DECISION MAKING IN HEALTH EDUCATION

by Gus T. Dalis and Ben B. Strasser

Acknowledgments

First, the authors would like to say "Thanks" to the Lane County Schools in Eugene, Oregon, because a workshop we did for them in 1969 was the stimulus that got our work in the area of values going strong. Second, special acknowledgment must be made for the continuing contribution of our partners in the Teaching Strategies Center, Dennis Loggins and Ray Cowan, in the refinement of our original ideas and the addition of new ones.

Finally, we must add that without the support of our Office and the interest of teachers of school districts in Los Angeles County who have participated, and continue to participate, in our four-day Values Awareness Teaching Strategy Workshop, the Values Awareness Teaching Strategy would probably have gone no further than a one-time inservice program.

Foreword

Wasn't there a time for all of us when the term "value" elicited a set of collective beliefs which evolved from tradition, custom, societal pressure, or moral laws? Unanimity was an adequate determinant of values while consequences often served as a deterrent. But in less than the past two decades when social institutions and social inventions were subjected to open criticisms — some deserving and others self-serving — many steadfast values appear to have toppled from their pinnacle of righteousness. This spillage built societal momentum for the examination, clarification, and exploration of values. Any mystical or other philosophical underpinnings that may have existed began to give way for some to pragmatic sanctions. Rather than professed values giving direction to behavior, one's behavior seemed as the reference point for value formation. This is not to say that the upheaval was universal, but academe provided a fertile ground for nourishing the value-free dialogue. Out of this background there is now a renewed concern for the development of a rationale for values education. The pendulum is moving toward a position in which educational institutions are being charged with the responsibility to "set standards and teach values." A recent NASSP-USOE Conference focused on the need for values education in schools along with a specific recommendation for inservice education of staff.

The plethora of discourse about values education in print, from the speaker's podium, and in workshop settings, give no evidence of decreasing concern about this issue. Can values be taught or can we only teach toward values? Should teaching be value-free? Can it be? Is there a role for decision making in the valuing process?

What is unique about this book that makes it distinctive among the many others that have already appeared in print or are among forthcoming publications? One of the most significant and insightful contributions of this book is that the authors distinguish between a *value statement*, such as "I prefer...", and a *value*, such as "I prefer...for the following reasons." Thus, it becomes evident that, although there may be consensus of preferences about a given object, idea or ideology, the *underlying reasons* for the preference may be many and varied. It is the latter, "the reasons for or why" which reflect our values and which sets the theme for this new perspective on values and the decision-making process.

Throughout the pages of this book, the reader will find a systematic presentation of the concept of values; decision making within the context of the DALSTRA model; six teaching strategies for health education; guidelines for selecting and building the appropriate teaching strategy, with particular emphasis on values awareness; teaching and student behaviors related to values awareness teaching; and, evaluating a value awareness lesson.

The presentation of each section in this book is replete with examples with which teachers and students can readily identify. These illustrations are used to reinforce the theoretical constructs discussed and provoke the reader's thinking about other real life decisions and the corresponding dimensions of value awareness.

The format of the text is refreshing; a pleasing alternative to the usual pages of conventional narrative style. The change of pace includes some narrative, simple diagrams, a few more complex models, and pages strategically placed that are devoted to a synthesis of ideas in the form of principles and guidelines.

Although the title of the book would indicate it is focused on health education, the theoretical framework is applicable to any subject matter area. The examples from health education are related to contemporary issues of concern to all individuals. Professional personnel with teaching responsibilities in health, nursing and medical education, allied health, as well as supervisors, curriculum coordinators, administrators, and others will find the mix of theory and application adaptable for a variety of teaching/learning environments such as the classroom, laboratory, workshop, community group meetings, and institute settings.

The authors are eminently qualified in the areas of teaching, consulting, and supervision, as both are consultants in the office of the Superintendent of the Los Angeles County Schools. This volume is a culmination of more than a decade of their thinking, working, writing, and speaking on the subjects of teaching strategies, decision making, and values awareness throughout this country and in other parts of the world. But most important, the real world of the classroom is the source of their credibility.

Elena M. Sliepcevich
Professor, Department of Health Education
Professor, School of Medicine
Southern Illinois University
Carbondale, Illinois

(formerly Director, School Health
Education Study, Washington, D.C.)

Table of Contents

1

An Emerging Thrust of Health Education

It's not a question of whether values influence health-related decision making or not, but rather what particular values influence those decisions as they are made.

It has been said that health, like sleep, is not appreciated until it is interrupted. What does it take to get people to take their health seriously? How many people realize that many of the day-to-day decisions they make have a significant influence on their well-being? In some instances, the impact of these decisions may be felt immediately, while more frequently, the results may not be realized until some time later. Too often, too little attention is given to the many daily health-related decisions that confront individuals. Sometimes this is so because of indifference. At other times, it may happen because of ignorance. In many instances, indepth consideration is given to health-related decisions only in retrospect, after one's health has been interrupted.

Since ancient times, mankind has been concerned about preserving health. Health education is the means whereby individuals, families, and communities gain those insights and skills necessary to protect and promote their well-being. Early attempts at formal health education centered on topics such as diet, cleanliness, and disease control.[1] In addition to these three issues, what additional content makes up the present discipline of health education? This same question asked of the physics teacher so as to ascertain the make up of physics might yield a response such as, "Physics centers on fundamental concepts of time, space, matter, light, motion, electricity,

1

and the physics of the atom."[2] And, the biology teacher might respond with, "changes of living things through time (evolution), diversity of type and unity of pattern of living things, genetic community of life, biological roots of behavior, complementarity of organisms and environment, complementarity of structure and function, regulation and homeostasis, science as inquiry, and the history of biological concepts."[2]

How does the health educator respond to a request about what students should study in health education? Over the past centuries, innovations in thought, inventions, advances in science and technology, industrialization, technology, population increases, urbanization, and ever increasing insights into well-being have led to the expansion of the body of knowledge related to health. Complexities of living today require the health educator to deal with a body of health knowledge and skills far beyond diet, cleanliness, and disease control. This expanded body of knowledge is essential if health education is going to help make it possible for the individual to realize the fullest potential for self, family, and the various communities of which each person will be a part.

Perhaps the best way to gain insight into what comprises the discipline of health education in the mid-1970s is to review the major concepts or strands dealt with in selected programs of health education across the country. Several states along with a national health curriculum study have prepared documents designed to communicate the breadth and scope of their programs in health education. What follows is an outline of the content of the health education programs as set forth by the States of California, Illinois, New York and the School Health Education Study Curriculum Project.

Through the 1972 "Framework for Health Instruction in California Public Schools, Kindergarten Through Grade Twelve," the California State Department of Education recommends that the following be dealt with in health education classes:

- Consumer health.
- Mental — emotional health.
- Drug use and misuse.
- Family health.
- Oral health, vision, and hearing.
- Nutrition.
- Exercise, rest, and posture.
- Diseases and disorders.
- Environmental health hazards.
- Community health resources.

A review of the "School Code of Illinois" outlines the major educational areas that should be dealt with in comprehensive health education programs in that state. These areas are:

- Human ecology and health.
- Human growth and development.
- Prevention and control of disease.
- Public and environmental health.
- Consumer health.
- Safety education and disaster survival.
- Mental health and illness.
- Personal health habits.
- Alcohol.
- Drug use and misuse.
- Tobacco.
- Nutrition.
- Dental health.

The "Prototype Curriculum Materials for Elementary and Secondary Grades: Health," developed by the University of the State of New York and the State Education Department, recommend the following strands be taught:

1. Physical Health, including health status, nutrition sensory perception, dental health, and disease prevention and control.
2. Sociological Health Problems, including smoking and health, alcohol education, and drugs and narcotic education.
3. Mental Health, including personality development, sexuality and family life education.
4. Environmental and Community Health, including environmental and public health, world health, ecology and epidemiology of health, and consumer health.
5. Education for Survival, including safety and first aid, and survival education.

In 1967, a national curriculum project, the School Health Education Study, produced, "Health Education: A Conceptual Approach to Curriculum Design." This publication outlined the following concepts for a comprehensive curriculum in health education:

- Growth and development influences and is influenced by the structure and functioning of the individual.
- Growing and developing follows a predictable sequence, yet is unique for each individual.
- Protection and promotion of health is an individual, community, and international responsibility.
- The potential for hazards and accidents exists, whatever the environment.

- There are reciprocal relationships involving man, disease, and environment.
- The family serves to perpetuate man and to fulfill certain health needs.
- Personal health practices are affected by a complexity of forces, often conflicting.
- Utilization of health information, products and services is guided by values and perceptions.
- Use of substances that modify mood and behavior arises from a variety of motivations.
- Food selection and eating patterns are determined by physical, social, mental, economic, and cultural factors.

Clearly, while including concerns of earlier years, health education of the late 1960s and early 1970s went far beyond the areas of diet, cleanliness, and disease control.

Without a doubt, the most important focus of health education is to sharpen the individual's ability to use health concepts taught as they make an ever widening array of health-related decisions that have a positive effect on his or her over-all well-being. This purpose is supported easily by reviewing current literature in health education. For example, the Bureau of Health Education, established in 1974 under the authority of the Secretary of Health, Education and Welfare, adopted the following definition of health education [3]:

> A process with intellectual, psychological and social dimensions relating the activities which increase the abilities of people to make informed decisions affecting their personal, family and community well-being.

In 1975, the Committee to Develop a Statement of Philosophy for Health Education, of the Association for the Advancement of Health Education, specified several alternatives as foci for health education. One of these alternatives, "Educate people to make wise decisions..." clearly suggests the need for decision making in health education. Interestingly, many of the other alternatives set forth by this group reinforce this position. [4]

In the sixth edition of *Health Education,* Russell shares the observation that:

> The task of the school — and of health education — is to encourage each learner to interact with some new information, ideas and concepts, and some new ways of learning so that future life interacting will be from a wide base, and one's decisions can be the results of a broader range of considerations. [5]

The decision making thrust of health education is indelible. While an emphasis on decision making is becoming a more significant element of many present day health education programs, a review of many school health education programs reveals that teachers attempt to influence their student's decision making by:

- Overt preaching about what is good.
- Appeals to morality.
- Using scare tactics that emphasize dangers of poor decisions.
- Presenting facts based upon scientific studies and research.
- Informing students about the range of health problems they are confronted with.
- Suggesting alternative ways of responding to health-related problems.

While some of these approaches may work with some students, more often than not, they yield unpredictable and undesired outcomes. Furthermore, these approaches overlook the act of making decisions. As a result, the emphasis of instruction is on giving the students the teacher's solutions rather than on decision-making abilities. While relevant facts and a knowledge of alternatives is fundamental in decision making, to properly consider alternatives related to matters of health the individual needs to be aware of his or her motives and values. Consider the following statement adopted by the Governing Council of the American Public Health Association [6]:

Education for and about health is not synonymous with information (acquisition). Education is concerned with behavior — a composite of what an individual knows, senses and values and of what one does and practices.

The central thrust of health education has to be comprehensive in scope of content and process. That is, health education needs to acquaint individuals with the range of health concepts related to daily life in a complex society. In addition, health education needs to focus on helping individuals develop and sharpen their decision-making capabilities so that interruptions to their health can be minimized.

To foster decision making, health education must go beyond helping individuals acquire health information, develop basic health concepts, and sharpen critical intellectual skills. Health education must also focus on helping students gain insight into themselves and recognize how their values affect the multitude of daily health-related decisions they make. By so doing, health education can contribute to the shift from unskilled decision makers — those who look upon the call for a decision as just another nagging trauma of living — to skilled decision makers — those who know what's involved in decision making, who have confidence in their ability to make a decision, and who view the call for a decision as a challenge and integral element of zestful living.

2

A Concept of Value
for the Classroom

For any teaching strategy in values to be effective it must be rooted in a concept of value that makes sense to students and teachers alike.

A fundamental purpose of education is to foster thoughtful, rational, and responsible decision making. One basis for such decision making is an individual's values. However, without a concept of value, it is difficult for someone to know what their values are, no less use them as a base for judgments and actions. Any educational program that focuses on decision making and values must, therefore, be rooted in a concept of value that works for both students and teachers.

Value Defined

V   *a preferred or*
A   *important quality,*
L   *characteristic,*
U   *attribute, or*
E   *property*

Values range in significance from those that serve as a moral or ethical guide people use to give direction and meaning to their lives such as...

HONOR	FREEDOM
RESPECTFUL	HONESTY
RELIABLE	SELF-RESPECT
DISCIPLINED	WISDOM
LOGICAL	RESPONSIBLE
OBEDIENT	EQUALITY
THOUGHTFUL	TRUSTWORTHY

. . . . to those which serve as a base for decision making about
routine, run-of-the-mill matters of living
  functional, effective, efficient, capable, economical, friendly,
imaginative, independent, complete, disposable, nonpolluting,
utilitarian, reusable, practical, unique, free, attractive,
priceless, sturdy, and so on.
  Values connote that which has worth. Since values are preferred
qualities, characteristics, attributes, or properties considered to reflect
intrinsic or enduring excellence by an individual or group, it is obvious
that. . .

V	*are*
A	*usually*
L	*stated*
U	*in*
E	*positive*
S	*terms*

Using Values

V	*serve as*
A	*a base for*
L	*decisions,*
U	*actions*
E	*or*
S	*judgments*

  Consider the statement, *Of the three health plans available to me,
I like the Red Circle Health Plan best because you are free to choose
your own physician.* The value utilized in making this judgment is,
freedom to choose your own physician. The judgment that the Red
Circle Health Plan is "best" is consistent with this value.
Obviously a rational decision is also based on data. Data in this case
is information available about whether or not the Red Circle Health
Plan does indeed allow subscribers to select their own physician.
  While the foregoing definition and examples of values may
suggest that there is a one-to-one relationship between an individual's
values and his judgments, actions, and decisions, life is usually more
complex than that. Any judgment, action, or decision is usually the
result of an interplay among several values as well as data. Frequently
such values may even be in conflict.
  Other values which may influence an individual's judgment about
the Red Circle Health Plan might include:

Values	Data
Expediency	just a signature on the line and you're a member;
Promptness	they are quick to reimburse the member whenever personal funds may have been expended for a physician or for medication;
Simplicity	a claim form is used that requires only the member's signature, the dates of the expenditure, and the physician's signature;
Economy	however, the Red Circle Health Plan costs more than all of the other health plans available.

Whether any or all of the above values influence people's judgment about a particular health plan depends upon what they know about the health plans, what they're looking for in a health plan, and the data they are able to generate about those health plans. Knowledge of their values enables people to identify what data they need to determine the degree to which their values are represented in a particular choice.

Discussing Values

Following are two comments about health plans:

In my view, the Red Circle Health Plan is the best one for me.

Some of my values about health plans are that they are economical, comprehensive, and give you the freedom to choose your own physician.

Both comments are responses to a question. The first is a response to the question, *Which health plan do you like?* It is a value judgment. The second comment is a response to the question, *What are your values about health plans?* It is a value statement.

To communicate values directly in a way that no room for "guestimates" is left for the listener, it is important that the individual let others know by labeling the values reported and indicating to what those values apply. With reference to the value statement given earlier, the phrase, "Some of my values..." lets others know they're listening to a value statement, "...about health plans..." indicates what the values are applied to, and "...economical, ..." are the actual values cited. Thus, a value statement is:

V	*a set of*
A	*words which,*
L	*(1) specify*
U	*what the*
E	*value is;*
S	*(2) label*
T	*the value as*
A	*such; and*
T	*(3) specify*
E	*the subject*
M	*of the value;*
E	*that to which*
N	*the value*
T	*is applied.*

While value statements usually include these three elements, they may occur in any sequence.

Some of my values about health plans are that they are economical, comprehensive, and give you the freedom to choose your own physician.

Promptness of service is one of my values about a health plan.

When considering which health plan to join, one of my values is convenience; that is, it is close to my home and easy to get in to see the physician.

It is important to note that even though many of the things people do and say are based on their values, it is only through a value statement that people communicate values directly. Since value judgments communicate only how people may feel about someone, something, or some place, the values which underlie these judgments are left to speculation. It is not unusual to find several people who agree with a given value judgment, action, or decision, but who do so based on values which differ significantly from each other. And there are those who may not know what their values are, no less be able to communicate them effectively to others.

3

A Notion of Natural Values Development

Values aren't taught as a subject, they are learned as a result of ways the environment and the people in it respond to the growing child. Thus, feedback is the critical element in the development of an individual's value system.

Often as we participate in discussions about values, an unspoken message that seems to come across is that values are "things out there," all ordered in a guidebook with a title something like, *Rules to Live By.* In our view, such lists of values often have little significance. Rather, it is those values that live inside of people that are important — the special property of each individual.

What follows is a way of thinking about how an individual's values evolve from a rudimentary set of behavior patterns to what we call functional values. This development is organized into four levels. We refer to Level I as Developing Behavior Patterns: Pre-Values; Level II as Developing Behavior Standards: Intuitive Values; Level III as Developing Insight Into Behavior Standards: Awareness Values; and Level IV as Developing A Consistency Between Behavior and Values: Functional Values.

The movement of individuals through these levels is an unfolding process that closely parallels their physical, mental, and social development. Although the behavior of all normal children can be related to the first level of development, it does not necessarily follow that growing and developing carries with it the automatic movement through levels two and three, into level four. Perhaps this is because not all adults are actively concerned about their values or the values of others. Perhaps it is the fault of our educational system because work in the arena of values is not based on a concept of value that makes sense to our students. Perhaps it is due to an individual's intellectual capabilities or the environment in which he matures or both. And, there may be other reasons.

Level I

Development Behavior Patterns: Pre-Values

As the infant begins to interact with his immediate surroundings, he or she learns how that environment responds to him. For example, when the child crawls around on the living room floor and pushes the fuzzy ball, mother and father smile and offer him sounds of encouragement.

He gets the message: *This must be good.* On the other hand, he may invite sounds of displeasure or even a slap on the hand when he artfully throws a spoon full of food onto the kitchen floor; thus, the message: *That's not so good.*

Even his extra-human environment communicates such messages to him. When he pets the family cat, it makes a nice sound and may gently rub against him. On the other hand, to pull the cat's tail results in another kind of sound and perhaps even a scratch or two.

He also finds that to crawl around on the bed is soft and fun, but to try to crawl from the bed to the floor is another story.

All of these kinds of events offer the youngster some feedback about his behavior. Some things he does mean good news for him. Some mean bad news. Such good news and bad news facilitates the development of behavior patterns.

A behavior pattern is a specific behavior that is repeated under similar circumstances. *I should play carefully with Barbara's football,* is based on what has happened to him when he played with Barbara's football in the past. *I shouldn't hit Clyde,* is based on what has happened to him in the past when he did. *I ought to drink my milk,* is based on what Mother has said or done when milk has been placed before him at the table.

In growing from infancy to the world of the primary grades, the child's interactions with others broaden to include the kids in his class and school, his teachers, and other adults. He finds that these people also communicate *good* and *not-so-good* messages to him. This serves as more information for him about how others respond to what he does and does not do. As a result, his range of behavior patterns expands to accommodate his widening world. However, of all the feedback the child gets as he interacts with his environment, it is primarily the way other humans act and react that lay the foundations for his values.

Of course, because a child adopts a behavior pattern does not necessarily mean he will conform to it. If that were true, there would be no such thing as risk-taking! And, it does not necessarily mean that the child is able to verbalize these patterns of behavior. It does mean, however, that you can see evidence of them in the child's behavior as he interacts with others and with his environment.

Perhaps what is of greatest significance in these very early stages of development is that, while behavior patterns are not values, they serve as values for the young child. That is, they serve as a base for his decisions about how he interacts with others and things around him.

Level II

Developing Behavior Standards: Intuitive Values

For most young children, behavior patterns are all they need to deal with their world. As they mature, however, their increasing interactions with others results in an ever widening array of behavior patterns. To cope with the increasing number of behavior patterns, a new level of development may emerge. The individual conceptualizes and adopts behavior standards.

A behavior standard is a "rule for behaving" or a cultural or subcultural norm which speaks to a range of related situations. For example, such behavior patterns as: *I shouldn't break Jamie's toy car when I play with it; I shouldn't ride off the curb with Hilda's bicycle; I should take care of Caleb's dollhouse;* are generalized and may become a behavior standard such as: *I should be careful when using things that belong to other people.* As in the case of behavior patterns, behavior standards serve as "values" in the absence of conceptualized values.

Level III

Developing Insight into Behavior Standards: Awareness Values

There is little doubt that behavior patterns and behavior standards are an outgrowth of the values of the society or subculture of which one is a part. At the Awareness of Value Level, the individual is engaged both in developing a concept of value and in using that concept as a way to learn about himself and his culture. For example, at this level, the individual moves beyond a behavior standard such as: *I should be careful when using things that belong to other people,* to the identification of a value that undergirds this standard such as: *consideration for the property of others.*

An individual may develop a concept of value in many different ways. These ways may range from adopting "textbook" definition on the one hand, to intuiting a concept of value for himself. With an understanding of a concept of value, he may become aware of his values through social dialogue or through reflective thinking. Someone else may make observations about what they believe his values to be by drawing inferences from what he says and does. Of course, the individual may accept or reject such comments. Or, he can utilize a process whereby he is able to surface his values for himself.

Actually, becoming aware of one's own values seldom occurs as a result of one or the other of these approaches alone. Some values are best surfaced through social dialogue while some values are best surfaced by the individual for himself. This latter type process involves reflective thinking and evolves from the question, *What is important to me about....?* It is also based on the individual's ability to infer values from and relate them to actions, decisions, and judgments.

Level IV

Developing a Consistency Between Behavior and Values: Functional Values

At this level of development, an individual has gone far beyond using behavior standards as a base for his behavior alone. His efforts at the Awareness Level have yielded him an operational concept of value and the ability to use it. As a result, he moves to the Functional Level at which he either knows what his priority values are or he is able to surface the values that influence his action, judgment, or decision for a given issue. In addition, he is more able to consciously anticipate and respond to situations in which there is a potential for values conflict. He also recognizes the role of both values and data and the interrelationship between them as they influence his decisions, actions, and judgments.

Societal values and the need for their continuing examination and reordering become a major concern for the individual at this level. This concern manifests itself in dialogue about the values of society with special attention to how conditions act on and influence a society's current prioritization of values. He is able, ready, and willing to make a case for values he considers essential to an effective society. He consciously behaves consistent with such values and may try to encourage others to do so as well.

The Effect of Feedback on Values
Reinforcement and Modification

So far, a process whereby individuals develop values from childhood to adulthood has been discussed. However, not all of a child's emerging values are what his or her parents or others would like them to be. Perhaps because of their egocentric orientation, some individual's values grow irrespective of the fact that those values may foster actions that yield negative consequences for them or others. Yet, some time later, the same individual may behave quite differently in a similar situation. For example, consider the nine year old who "forgets" to brush his teeth for weeks on end, while at age 17, the same individual brushes his teeth twice a day regularly.

Since one's values are a base for decisions about actions, a change in behavior suggests either that the individual's values have changed or that his values priorities have changed.

Note the two ways of explaining this same phenomenon: the individual's values changed, or his values priorities changed. One view holds that a given value may be modified or discarded, to be replaced by another value. The second view takes the position that all people hold essentially the same values. It is rather a question of which of those values are used as a base for the specific decision to be made. Which view we use is immaterial. What is of significance is that either people's values or values priorities change overtime. The issue of concern to educators is, *What happened to bring about that change?*

In our view, the same process that influenced the development of the value in the first place may serve to reinforce an individual's value or stimulate the reconsideration of a value — namely, values feedback.

Earlier we described how infants get *good* and *not-so-good* messages about their behavior from their environment. All such messages are feedback for the individual — data for him in relation to how his actions made him and others feel. An individual may get direct or vicarious feedback about his behavior or about his values. Direct feedback about behavior happens as an individual behaves and (1) is sensitive to his own responses to what he did, and/or (2) observes the responses of others to him. For example, consider the situation in which Creighton has had four or five drinks at a party after a school dance. He gets direct feedback about his behavior both as he feels "shaky" and as he overhears some of his friends commenting about his unstable condition. It is personal feedback for him. In essence, living is behaving, and everytime an individual behaves he has an opportunity to get direct feedback about his behavior if he is sensitive to it.

Fortunately, human beings do not have to experience everything for themselves to learn. The world is also rich with opportunities to observe the behavior of others. We refer to this as vicarious feedback, or social learning. Vicarious feedback about behavior happens as an individual observes both the behavior of someone else and the effects of that behavior. By relating the two, he gains some insight into how others might respond to him in a similar situation. Again, let us consider the situation in which Creighton has had four or five drinks at a party. An observer may be sensitive to his own reactions to Creighton's behavior and/or to the responses of others to him. Vicarious feedback about behavior may also happen as a result of reading an article or a book, watching films, gossiping over the back fence or participating in group discussions, role playing, role reversal situations, or other group dynamic activities.

When an individual has a concept of value, he may also utilize direct or vicarious feedback about his values rather than about his behavior alone. Direct values feedback may happen in a social setting as an individual responds with agreement or disagreement. It may happen as an individual asks others about what their values are. He then relates what he hears to his values. Vicarious values feedback may happen for an individual as he observes how others respond to someone who has reported one of their values. Both direct or vicarious feedback may be utilized by individuals no matter their level of values development. For individuals at the Pre-Values or Intuitive Values levels, the feedback is related to behavior patterns or behavior standards respectively. However, because individuals at the Awareness of Values and Functional Values levels have a concept of value, they are able to go one step further with their feedback; they can also relate the feedback about behavior to the values which underlie that behavior. Consequently, whether direct or vicarious feedback serves as feedback about behavior patterns, behavior standards, or values, depends primarily on the individual's level of values development. Figure 1 summarizes ways in which feedback may reinforce one's values or stimulate the reexamination of them.

FIGURE 1

FEEDBACK AND VALUES REINFORCEMENT

Values reinforcement takes place as

people perceive that their:

* Actions which are consistent with their
  values yield positive outcomes

* Values are consistent with those
  they respect or admire

* Values are consistent with
  the values of their culture

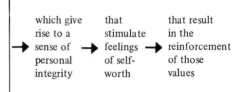

which give rise to a sense of personal integrity → that stimulate feelings of self-worth → that result in the reinforcement of those values

FEEDBACK AND THE NEED FOR VALUES MODIFICATION

Values modification may be stimulated
as people perceive that their:

* Actions which are consistent with their
  values yield negative outcomes

* Values are inconsistent with the values
  of those they respect or admire

* Values are inconsistent with the values
  of their culture

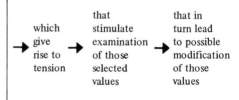

which give rise to tension → that stimulate examination of those selected values → that in turn lead to possible modification of those values

4

Decision Making and Health Education

The opportunity to make a decision isn't a problem or headache, it's a chance to exercise some control over your life.

Decision Making — What's Missing?

An obvious goal of school health education is to improve the quality of students' health. While there are some aspects of an individual's health over which he or she may have no control, there is no doubt that a person can exert a significant impact on his or her overall well-being. Ultimately, this impact is exerted through the range of health-related choices made and implemented throughout day-to-day living. Because the goal of school health education is to improve the quality of students' health, it follows that the central thrust of health education is toward exerting a positive influence on that moment of impact — the act of decision making.

In the belief that data is the base for all decision making, health instruction has historically emphasized giving students data and information health educators feel is fundamental to making and implementing health-related decisions. The assumption is that if teachers teach their students the necessary concept and data, the students will make "good" decisions. Working with concepts and data also necessitates the need for students to be able to generate, evaluate, and organize data on their own. As a result, most health education programs also stress the development of these intellectual abilities.

Despite the fact that more and new facts and concepts continue to be added to the health education curriculum in the hopes that health education can be more effective, it is clear that the outcomes of such programs continue to fall far short of our expectations. Teachers find that their students still make health-related decisions that have

19

negative effects on their well-being. Perhaps this is so because we are not giving the students enough data and information. Perhaps this is so because students are just unable to learn the masses of data that they will need for effective decision making throughout their lives. Or, perhaps the outcomes of current health education programs fall short of our expectations; in dealing with concepts, data, and data generating, data evaluating, and data organizing skills alone, to expect that we are facilitating the development of students as rational decision makers, is a false hope.

Decision Making as Problem Solving

It may be that one source of the disappointments health educators experience lies in the concept of decision making being taught. Or it might be that the way decision making is being taught is in need of some thinking.

Decision making is the act of trying to find a suitable solution for a certain kind of problem. Usually the solution sought is a course of action to be implemented, *to decide what should be done about,* or to make a value judgment, *to decide if something is good or bad, whether to agree or disagree, etc.* Decision making in the area of health education centers on such issues as:

- What foods should (and shouldn't) I eat?
- What kind of physical activity should I engage in?
- What should I do for my cold?
- Should I smoke?
- What kinds of immunization should I get?
- How should I vote on the fluoridation issue?
- What should I do if I drink and have to get somewhere that requires driving?
- How frequently should I visit my physician and dentist for a checkup?
- Should I (we) use family planning measures?
- What factors should I consider before using any nonprescription medicines?
- Should I experiment with pot?
- What should I do when I feel awkward in a group?

While decision making is problem solving, not all problem solving is decision making. Inquiring is a way of solving some other kinds of problems. In inquiring, people use a network of inquiry processes in search of "value-free" solutions, theories or explanations.* In the area of health education, inquiry invites students to build solutions for problems such as:

* Despite the abundance of a variety of relatively inexpensive foods available in the United States, why are there so many people who suffer from poor nutrition?

* Even though there are known VD prevention measures, why is the incidence of gonorrhea and syphilis infections increasing at an alarming rate?

* Why is it that more than two billion dollars a year is spent in the United States for fake remedies and quack cures for illness?

In reviewing decision making and inquiry as two kinds of problem solving, it is important to highlight a significant difference between them. Theories or explanations in inquiry are judged not on how well someone likes them, but rather on how well they fit with the data available. In inquiry, data "rules" as the prime base to evaluate a theory. Imagine, for example, that an individual or group spends considerable time and energy to develop an explanation for the current surge in the occurrence of venereal diseases. As a result of this effort, they report a theory they have developed which is consistent with their data. If their theory is a good one, it should probably also fit with data others may generate or have generated in similar inquiries. A theory or explanation which was developed through honest inquiry and which is viewed as good by one person is generally viewed as good by other people as well. If the data fits with the theory or explanation, it fits. If the data does not fit with the theory for one person, the same data probably would not fit when other people evaluate that theory. The intent of inquiry, therefore, is to attempt to produce "individual proof" solutions by using inquiry processes that yield theories or solutions as value free as humanly possible.

As value free as inquiry is intended to be, decision making is just the opposite. While data are also utilized in making decisions, decision making centers on individual or group values, depending on whether individual or group decision making is involved. Data serves as evidence the decision maker uses to determine the degree to which his or her priority values are represented in the alternative solutions considered. While theories or explanations developed through inquiry are intended to be "true for all," the product of decision making is intended to be appropriate primarily for the decision maker. Whether others like the solution or not is of a lesser concern.

For a detailed discussion of inquiry, see Strasser, et al: Teaching Toward Inquiry. Schools for the 70's Action Series, National Education Association, Washington, D.C., 1971.

A (One) Model of Decision Making

What follows is one way of thinking about the act of decision making. There are two reasons why previously available models of decision making were felt inadequate. First, while several of these models allude to values as influencing decision making, the way that this influence is felt is not outlined. The second reason it was necessary to develop a model of decision making is that other models dealt only with the act of making very involved, important or "rational" decisions. Other ways of making life's less critical or less significant decisions are ignored. It is as though one does not make a decision unless it is a very significant one. The purpose of the Model of Decision Making presented here (Figure 2) is to account for these two shortcomings. The influence of values is outlined and the model accounts for the variety of ways people make decisions in their day-to-day lives.

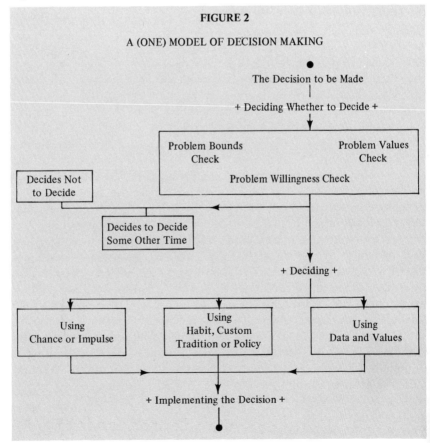

FIGURE 2

A (ONE) MODEL OF DECISION MAKING

This model is not intended to be a highly detailed view of decision making nor is it intended to outline how decisions should be made. Rather, it is a descriptive statement about different ways individuals or groups respond to different kinds of decision-making problems they encounter. Furthermore, while the model may seem to be highly academic in written form, we emphasize that these processes happen many times throughout the day — most frequently at the intuitive level.

In this model, decision making is treated in two phases. Phase I centers on the decision-making antecedents and Phase II describes three modes of decision making. The decision-making antecedents are discussed first — deciding whether to decide and how to decide. Then, three ways of making decisions are outlined: the Chance or Impulse Mode of Decision Making; the Habit, Custom, Tradition or Policy Mode of Decision Making; and the Data and Values Mode of Decision Making.

Once a decision is made, if the decision involves doing something, that action must be implemented using whatever means is appropriate. Since the act of implementing a decision is beyond the act of decision making, we have chosen not to include a discussion of ways decisions may be implemented in this material.

Deciding Whether to Decide: The Decision-Making Antecedents

Decision making has been defined earlier as the act of identifying and selecting a solution for a problem. Before actual decision making is initiated, however, some other kinds of things happen. Obviously, the individual or group must first be aware of the need to decide; she or he must be aware of the problem. Then, three other issues emerge. In responding to questions such as, *How important is it that the problem be solved?* and/or *How urgent is the problem?* the individual is doing a PROBLEM VALUES CHECK. It is one way of determining how significant the problem is for the individual as he or she relates the problem to his or her values.

Depending on the problem, thought may also be given to the question, *What constraints act on a successful solution for the problem?* Doing so is referred to as doing a PROBLEM BOUNDS CHECK. It centers on finding out about the nature of the problem itself which is necessary if a successful solution is to be found and implemented. Finally, the individual may give thought to questions such as, *Do I have to or want to respond to the problem? Am I ready and willing to respond to the problem?* In this case, the decision maker considers his or her own feelings about the decision to be made. This is referred to as a PROBLEM WILLINGNESS CHECK.

As an outgrowth of these decision-making antecedents, that may be done in any sequence, the individual may decide not to decide, or to decide at some other time.

On the other hand, the individual may feel the problem needs attention and the act of decision making is initiated. Since there are different ways the decision may be made, the responses to the PROBLEM VALUES CHECK, the PROBLEM BOUNDS CHECK and the PROBLEM WILLINGNESS CHECK serve as the bases from which the specific way of making the decision is determined. For example, given a problem determined to be relatively unimportant to the individual with relatively few constraints that bear on a successful solution and for which the individual does not have to respond, the Chance or Impulse Mode of Decision Making may be utilized.

Before turning to a discussion of these three modes of decision making, we note that by commenting about the decision-making antecedents we are not suggesting that all decision making should be a systematic and highly intellectual process. Nothing could be further from the truth. In most individual decision making, these antecedents usually happen at the intuitive or subconscious level — almost in the twinkling of an eye. In group decision making they are usually treated in a more deliberate and/or systematic way.

Making Decisions in Different Ways

The kinds of health-related decisions people make range from the incidental matters like, *What kind of bath soap should I buy?* to issues of more significance such as, *What immunizations should I have?*

Some decisions are easy because they deal with incidental matters. Other decisions are more difficult because they are ways people respond with issues of greater significance to them. Because the kinds of decisions people make range from the incidental to the significant, the ways people make decisions also differ. Some decisions are made by using chance or impulse to decide. Some decisions are made by referring to habit, custom, tradition, or a policy for a solution. That is all that is necessary in these cases. Some decisions, on the other hand, involve the more complex processes of explicating one's values relative to the decision to be made and generating data about the alternative solutions. This data and values mode of decision making may take from moments to days.

While these three ways of making decisions range in complexity, one way of deciding is not necessarily better than the others. Rather, it is a question of which decision-making mode is most appropriate for the decision to be made.

As each of these decision-making modes is reviewed in the material that follows, they are discussed by relating each mode to three basic elements common to all decision making (Figure 3).

While we have listed these three elements of each decision-making mode in what may appear to be a recommended sequence, it must be emphasized that people are creative thinkers. There are an infinite variety of ways these three elements may be implemented. For example, an individual may initiate and continue the "search" until several solutions are identified. Then the solutions may be "checked." In other instances, one solution may be identified, then checked. If it is found wanting, another solution may be sought, and so on. Even though there is individual variety in the way decisions are made, however, there is a recognizable progression from Search, to Check, to Select, which can be identified in the analysis of any decision made.

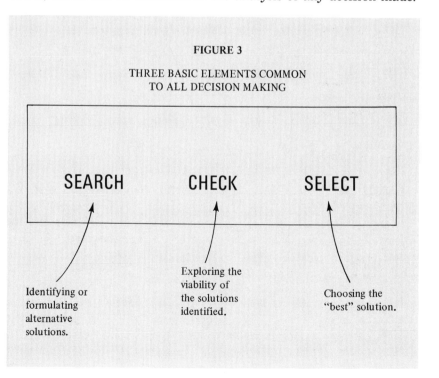

FIGURE 3

THREE BASIC ELEMENTS COMMON
TO ALL DECISION MAKING

SEARCH   CHECK   SELECT

Identifying or formulating alternative solutions.

Exploring the viability of the solutions identified.

Choosing the "best" solution.

Using Chance or Impulse to Decide

In some instances a person may find it necessary to make a decision about an issue that may not be very important to him or very significant in his life. Or, it may be that while the issue is important, she or he feels it is impossible to exert any real influence on the outcome. There may also be occasions in which either an individual has only a very limited time to decide, or the data needed in order to make a more systematic decision is not available. As a result, the decision may be made by chance or impulse.

Utilizing this way of making decisions involves selecting a solution by flipping a coin or by letting events take their course without intervention. Or, the individual (or group) may just pick a solution because it "feels okay" or "seems okay." Unquestionably, deciding by chance or impulse is the least complex way of making a decision.

Of course, since one's values are a prime base for any decision making, values are involved in this mode, though indirectly. That is, to make a decision by chance suggests that the outcome was not very significant as far as the individual's values are concerned. Or selecting a solution because it "feels okay" or "seems okay" suggests that the solution has passed an intuitive values check.

FIGURE 4

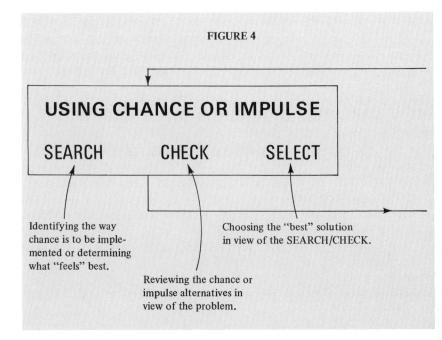

USING CHANCE OR IMPULSE

SEARCH   CHECK   SELECT

Identifying the way chance is to be implemented or determining what "feels" best.

Choosing the "best" solution in view of the SEARCH/CHECK.

Reviewing the chance or impulse alternatives in view of the problem.

When reviewed in terms of the search, check, and select elements of decision making, the Chance-Impulse way of making decisions seems to be least discrete in terms of the processes used. Emphasis of the search in Chance or Impulse decision making is directed toward selecting what way chance will be implemented or what feels best. The "check" is little more than a review of the chance or impulse considered in relation to the problem significance. This review is then followed by selecting the particular way to implement chance or that impulse solution that seems most appropriate (Figure 4).

There is no doubt that the Chance or Impulse way of making decisions is probably used more frequently than either of the other decision-making modes — and rightly so. It is doubtful that anyone could hold on to his or her sanity if all of the hundreds of decisions made during the day were given the kinds of attention characteristic of the other more complex ways of making decisions.

Using Habit, Custom, Tradition, or Policy to Decide

Another way people cope with the unending stream of decisions to be made is to utilize the Habit, Custom, Tradition, or Policy Mode of Decision Making. Generally, this way of making decisions is used when the decision to be made is of some significance to the individual and is a decision that has been and is to be faced repeatedly.

Making decisions by habit means using a solution again that has worked in the past in similar situations. Habit is a kind of ritualized behavior for an individual that happens almost without any deliberate thought.

Making decisions by custom refers to the use of some "norm" as a base to decide. *That's the way everybody does it.* Custom is a kind of informal rule of conduct or behavior. Tradition, on the other hand, is a more formalized or institutionalized kind of custom that is frequently defined by religious, social, family, group or cultural mores. Tradition is characterized as a custom that is handed down from generation to generation.

Policies, like habits, customs, or traditions, are solutions to problems before they arise. Policies are formally explicated "rules" that enable a group to decide about complicated problems systematically with relative ease and a minimum of time. Usually the need for a policy arises when a group finds itself having to make the same kind of decision again and again. A policy is formulated (using the Data and Values Mode of Decision Making to be discussed next) and the decision-making time is minimized.

When viewed in terms of the search, check, and select elements of decision making, these processes appear to be more discrete than in the Chance or Impulse Mode of Decision Making. The search involves a scanning of habits, customs, traditions, or policies believed to be relative to the problem. Once a search is made, a check is done to assure that the habit, custom, tradition, or policy identified will yield a valuable solution to the problem at hand. Finally, the specific solution to be implemented is selected (Figure 5).

While values do not appear to be directly involved in the Habit, Custom, Tradition, or Policy Mode of Decision Making, they are, nonetheless, very critically felt. Frequently, the habits, customs, traditions, or policies drawn on were originally developed through the third mode of decision making yet to be discussed — the Data and Values Mode of Decision Making.

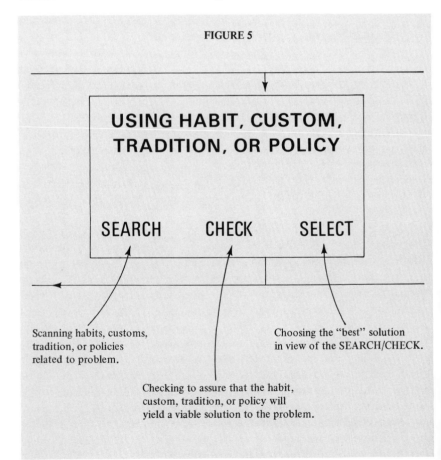

FIGURE 5

USING HABIT, CUSTOM, TRADITION, OR POLICY

SEARCH   CHECK   SELECT

Scanning habits, customs, tradition, or policies related to problem.

Choosing the "best" solution in view of the SEARCH/CHECK.

Checking to assure that the habit, custom, tradition, or policy will yield a viable solution to the problem.

Using Data and Values to Decide

The data and values way of making decisions is decidedly more considered, deliberate, and systematic than the other two modes of decision making previously discussed. Usually this mode of decision making is used because the problem is of great significance and there are no relevant habits, customs, traditions, or policies that will offer a good solution. With the exception of the role of values in the process to be outlined, this mode of decision making comes closest to the way other authors describe "rational" decision making.

As in the case of the other decision-making modes, the three elements: search, check, and select apply to this decision making as well. Data and Values decision making begins with a search for plausible, sensible solutions. To do so, the individual may brainstorm possibilities, glean ideas from others, use written materials or whatever. With some plausible solutions identified, those solutions are usually submitted to the three kinds of checks.

A probability check involves reviewing each plausible solution in terms of its chances for success. Usually this involves generating data from which predictions about potential success are made. As a result of a probability check, some solutions may be retained, others may be rejected and/or new alternatives may be sought.

In addition to a probability check, an impact check is used to analyze plausible solutions in terms of the effects implementing that solution may have on the individual, others affected and/or the environment. It may also include exploring other problems the proposed solution solves and new problems that may be created.

Another kind of check is what is referred to as a values check. In doing so, the plausible solutions are reviewed in the light of the individuals' values. While a values check may include explicating those values related to the decision to be made, the prime question dealt with is, *How do the plausible solutions and anticipated impact match with what's important to me — with my values?* The values check may then lead to data generating to determine the degree to which the individual's values are represented in the solutions being considered.

Values are crucial to this way of making decisions. In those instances where an individual (or group) either knows or is able to explicate his or her values related to the problem, he or she can utilize those values directly, deliberately, and openly in making the decision. In those instances in which the individual is unaware of his or her values, those values act at what might be called a subconscious level. That is, a plausible solution may be selected because it "feels right" without really understanding why it is so. One of the difficulties in using an intuitive values base to judge a plausible solution is that making the decision may be highly frustrating because there are competing values acting on the individual, but he or she is unaware of the source of the conflict and is, thereby, unable to respond to the real issue (Figure 6).

In view of these three kinds of checks which may take from moments to months, a plausible solution is selected; the decision is made. If none of the plausible solutions are found to be acceptable as a result of the check, other solutions may be sought. To the degree that all of the elements of the Data and Values Decision-Making Mode are dealt with thoughtfully, the greater are the chances that the decision will be successful. A decision made only on values or only on data is equally limited.

While there is little doubt that the Data and Values Mode of Decision Making is undoubtedly the most complex of the three modes presented, it does bear a close relationship to the Habit, Custom, Tradition, or Policy Mode of Decision Making. The data and values mode is used primarily to make new and significant decisions. If a similar decision is to be made at a later date, the same solution may be used again. Thus, a solution first developed through the data and values mode may become a solution which is later applied in the Habit, Custom, Tradition, or Policy Decision-Making Mode.

FIGURE 6

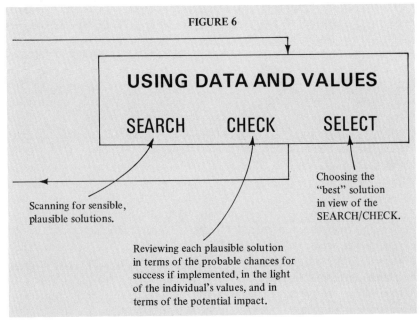

USING DATA AND VALUES

SEARCH   CHECK   SELECT

Scanning for sensible, plausible solutions.

Reviewing each plausible solution in terms of the probable chances for success if implemented, in the light of the individual's values, and in terms of the potential impact.

Choosing the "best" solution in view of the SEARCH/CHECK.

The Model of Decision Making —
Some Afterthoughts

Following is a potpourri of comments about the Model of Decision Making described. Some are disclaimers; some are added thoughts.

1. While at work on a problem, a person may change from one decision-making mode to another or abort all efforts to find a solution either because the problem itself or his or her understanding of it has changed.
2. The nature of human beings is such that an individual is usually working on many different problems at the same time, utilizing different decision-making modes, and with each decision to be made at a different place in the process.
3. Decision making may move from problem to solution freely or haltingly; it may take an instant or a lifetime and may be a pleasurable, anxious, or frustrating experience.
4. While three ways of making decisions are outlined in the model, it is important to emphasize that one way of making a decision is no better than another. It is a question of which decision-making mode is most appropriate to the decision to be made.
5. While a general linear movement though a sequence of decision-making processes may seem to be suggested in the Model, it is recognized that people usually move back and forth among the various search, check, and select processes as they work toward a decision.
6. Because of the way decision making is presented in the model, it may appear that the various decision-making processes involve only thinking. However, people may write down plausible solutions, predicted outcomes, possible impact on others, and so on, as a way to keep track of their thinking.
7. To the degree that an individual is aware of his values, data and values decision making can happen more systematically and deliberately.

Some Inferences for Instruction

At the beginning of this chapter, we suggested that one source of some of our disappointments with many present health education programs might be identified as the concept of decision making fundamental to such programs. When present health education programs are reviewed, it becomes clear that decision making is most frequently taught as though it is a purely data-based process. As a result, a major instructional emphasis in the classroom is on data and data generating, data validating, and data organizing processes. Certainly data are important in decision making. Without data, any decision could hardly be considered anything but irrational. Without special emphasis on the role of values in decision making, however, the central element of the decision-making process is missing. What decision making is all about — acting on one's values — is not dealt with. In addition to data, a major thrust of health education programs must be on developing the students' concept of value, on developing their ability to explicate their own values, on developing their ability to systematically infer the values of others, and on developing their awareness of their own values in relation to health-related issues and concerns.

With this Model of Decision Making in mind, it is possible to view health education from a different perspective. Since the way people exert an impact on their health is through the range of health-related choices they make as they live their lives, a major goal of health instruction is to shift the health related decisions students make by using the Chance or Impulse Mode of Decision Making to considered habits, customs, tradition, or policies or by using the Data and Values Decision-Making Mode.

Since making decisions using the Data and Values Decision-Making Mode rests on using data and concepts, information acquisition and concept development goals for instruction take on a new meaning. This decision-making mode also rests on the effective use of data generating, data organizing, and data processing skills. Thus, the need for skill development goals is also reinforced. In addition, because this mode of decision making also rests on the student's awareness of his or her own values, a values awareness goal for instruction becomes more significant than merely to help students gain some insight into what is important to them alone. It also suggests that, in addition to becoming informed about the different ways people make decisions, students also need opportunities to expand their repertoire of decision-making strategies if they are going to implement the Data and Values Decision-Making Mode more systematically, deliberately, and effectively.

5

Teaching and
Health Education

A central thrust of health education is to shift the mode of making health related decisions from chance-impulse to a data and values base.

Teaching Defined

Teaching is goal directed. Generally speaking, it involves someone who knows or who has particular skill working with someone who does not know or who does not have that skill. We call the person who "knows," the teacher, and the person(s) who does not, "students." When we talk about the act of teaching, therefore, we are talking about a system that includes a teacher or teachers who interact with a student or students. And, we see both students and teachers using their energies toward the eventual mastery of something to be learned. Their common purpose is to bridge the student's knowledge or skills gap.

This notion of teaching is age-free. That is, the teacher is defined by this function: someone who knows working with someone who does not know. In the broad sense, one child can function as the teacher for another as he helps his friend learn to ride a skate board. We refer to this as informal teaching.

Formal teaching, on the other hand, places certain responsibilities on the teacher-person. The teacher is assigned the position as a result of certification of some kind and the position carries with it the responsibility for students' learning as well as their personal welfare. Furthermore, formal teaching usually takes place over a specifically allocated period of time, in an assigned facility, and toward some lesson objective defined prior to instruction. This book is directed toward what we have called formal teaching.

Most of the time when teachers work with their students, they are working for specified lesson objectives. There are times, however, when teachers talk to their students about matters other than the substance of instruction — time when they may step out of their "teacher" relationship with the students and function in an adult friend role, in a counselor role, or in an advocate role. For example, a student may just want to talk to an adult about some of his interests or accomplishments, so that teacher may serve as a counselor in helping him surface his own feelings, his position, or alternatives open to him. Or, the student may have a problem with the school or community for which the teacher may act as an advocate in the student's behalf. Because of the significance of these kinds of issues in the lives of students, it is easy for teachers to become totally absorbed with their friend, counselor, and advocate functions. When this happens, there is the danger that they may lose sight of their primary responsibility — the implementation of the instructional objective they have for the students of their classroom.

Teaching Strategy Defined

If a group of visitors were to walk into any classroom where a lesson is in progress, they would see certain kinds of things going on. After observing awhile they would become aware of what the lesson is all about and where it is going. Soon they would see the lesson move through a developmental sequence from which they would get some sense of flow. They would find that the students are organized in certain ways and are using selected materials. And the students would be doing certain things (and not doing other possible things) as they participate in the lesson. The same is true of the teacher. That is, the effective teacher would be doing things consistent with what the lesson is all about and not doing some other things one might do that are inconsistent with the lesson. We suggest that the lesson flow, the way the classroom is organized, the materials being used, and what the students and teacher do during a lesson all happen because someone has decided that they should. The teacher has decided.

The teacher has made a decision about what the students will learn. Certainly, this decision might be directly or indirectly influenced by the students, or it may be modified during the lesson as the students participate. More frequently, the teacher's decision about what the students are to learn is based on district curriculum guides, textbooks, and so on. The teacher has also made a decision about the sequence the lesson is going to follow — where it will begin and how it will get where it is going. A lesson sequence may be used as recommended by the district and as modified by the teacher's perception of student needs. The teacher has also made some decision about how the students are to be organized and what materials they will use. Surely all of these decisions may also be open to the influence of the students — or the teacher may decide to let the students decide. But the teacher is still the person who is responsible, and accountable for these decisions.

The teacher also decides either explicitly or implicitly what the students are to do during the lesson. Certainly it is not that the teacher gives the students a continuing stream of moment-to-moment advice, but there are some general kinds of things the teacher expects the students to do during the lesson that will move them toward the desired lesson outcomes. For example, the teacher may expect the students to listen, to raise questions, to read, to observe, to discuss, to attend, to write, to participate in some kind of practice, to produce a given product, and so on, relative to some aspect of health. Finally, the teacher has made some decisions about what he is going to do and about his own behavior during the lesson.

What all of this boils down to is that, in effect, a lesson is the product of a set of professional decisions a teacher makes and which the students and teacher implement during the lesson. This is true whether these decisions are the result of deliberate and thoughtful planning or whether these decisions are the result of some flash of insight, a new idea to experiment with, or a spur-of-the-moment action. In light of what it is the students are to learn, the range of professional decisions to be made center on such instructional issues as:

- What are the learning steps and how are they to be sequenced?
- How will the students be organized?
- What materials will they use?
- What are the students to do as they come to grips with this particular learning task?
- What will the teacher do to initiate the lesson and to facilitate the student's growth toward the lesson objectives?

When the question, *"What is a teaching strategy?"* is raised, our response is:

Before the moment of teaching, a teaching strategy is a means to an end — a plan for action intended to make it possible for students to achieve a desired instructional outcome and which accounts for each of these aforementioned instructional issues.

During the moment of teaching, a teaching strategy is what is happening — what the teacher is doing and saying, what the students are doing and saying, the materials they are using, how they are organized, and so on.

After the lesson is over, the teaching strategy becomes the history of a human event.

An effective teaching strategy is one in which the answers to the instructional issues specified are precise, systematic, internally consistent, and which yields the intended outcome with students.

Teacher's Goals for Students

It is 3:30 as Ms. Jamison walks into the faculty lounge and joins her teacher friend, Ms. Johns, for a fresh cup of coffee. Once settled, Ms. Johns says: *What did you work on during your health lesson today, Prunella?*

Prunella responds with *We worked on trying to develop a concept of immunity. You know, it sure is....*

Seated nearby, Mr. Fodor joins the conversation by commenting that he is preparing to teach some lessons about local health services. *They sure need to know the kind of health services available to them in the community. Do either of you have any ideas I can use?*

And so discussions among faculty members go. There is talk about lessons intended to develop concepts, to develop skills, to give students information, and so on. Such language among teachers is useful to describe what we call *teacher's goal for their students.*

Concept development is one such goal for instruction. It is what the teacher sets out to accomplish with students. For example, a concept frequently taught in the area of drugs is: *Many factors and forces influence the use of substances that modify mood and behavior.*[1] Skill development is another such goal. For example, many teachers devote several lessons to developing the student's ability to analyze advertisements for health related products in order to assess the validity of the information presented. In addition to intellectual skills, health education may also include psychomotor skills such as developing the student's ability to correctly use a bandage to apply a compress to a wound.

Information acquisition is a third goal for health instruction. This teaching is intended to pass certain health information on to students, such as informing them about various health services available in the community. Providing facts about the harmful effects of smoking is another example of information to be provided for students. With recent emphasis on decision making as a primary thrust in health education, the arena of values awareness has gained increasing significance and attention as an instructional goal. Values awareness centers on helping students become aware of their own evolving system of health-related values and on developing student's ability to relate these values to their behavior. For example, the teacher may invite the students to discuss snack foods as a way of helping them surface some of their values about their nutrition practices. Yet another goal for health instruction focuses on human communication. Working toward this end, the teacher seeks to develop the student's ability to communicate effectively with others relative to a range of health issues.

Perhaps the primary goal of health instruction is to develop the student's ability to solve health-related problems and to make health-related decisions more rationally. In such lessons, for example, the teacher is concerned with helping students develop a range of processes useful to them in responding to such problems or decisions as, *How shall I vote on.....health issue? How do I respond to an invitation to drink liquor at a party? In what ways might I go about choosing a health plan?*

In general, most things teachers do in their health education classrooms can be classified as one of the six goals many teachers hold for their students. These six goals are: (1) concept development, (2) skill development, (3) information acquisition, (4) values awareness, (5) communication, and (6) the development of problem solving and/or decision-making strategies. Even a cursory review of these goals reveals that each is unique in terms of the expectations teachers hold for their students. It is one thing, for example, to expect students to recall the names of available community health services as an outgrowth of an information acquisition goal for health instruction. It is another thing, however, to expect students to make reasoned judgments about the effectiveness of the various community health services as an outgrowth of a skill development goal for instruction. In the first example, the students must listen or read and be able to recall the information at a later time. In the second example, the students must have sufficient opportunities to make reasoned judgments by locating and/or formulating criteria as a base for their evaluation, utilize the criteria by applying them to the data about the various health services they are evaluating, and make a judgment about the effectiveness of those health services that will stand up in the light of scrutiny by others.

It is apparent, therefore, that while all of the six kinds of goals mentioned for health education are indeed valid goals, students need to do different things to achieve those goals. Different goals require different lesson climates. Different goals require a different structure for the respective lessons; and, different goals require that the teacher do different things as she or he interacts with students. Thus, different goals for students require different teaching strategies.

6

Teaching Strategies for Health Education

One of the challenges for the teacher of health education is that the comprehensive curriculum centers on student objectives related to all six of the goals for students cited earlier. Since each of these goals is unique in terms of student expectations, each goal requires a different teaching strategy. Even though the primary purpose of this text is to present the Values Awareness Teaching Strategy in detail, it may be useful to present a brief overview of all six teaching strategies. In so doing, the Values Awareness Teaching Strategy will not be viewed as the answer to the present ills of health education but rather as one element of a comprehensive educational program.

We hasten to add that the six teaching strategies outlined are not the only teaching strategies teachers use in the classroom. They do represent those goals, however, that make up the mainstream of teaching. It should also be pointed out that not everything a teacher does, such as giving students a pretest at the beginning of a unit of work, is necessarily a teaching strategy.

Figure 7 is a list of the six goals for students along with the related teaching strategies to be discussed. In order to give the reader a mental picture of each of these teaching strategies, a descriptive paragraph is provided. In addition, the flow of a "typical" lesson is outlined by listing some characteristic elements of the teaching strategy. It is important to point out, however, that because of the students, the facilities, the teacher, time constraints, or the particular lesson objective, some lessons may be taught successfully by rearranging the sequence given or by deleting some of the lesson elements described; or, in some instances, the teacher might build in some additional lesson elements for the same reasons.

FIGURE 7

Teacher's Goals for Students	Related Teaching Strategies
● To acquire information about . . .	● Information Acquisition Teaching Strategy
● To develop concepts about . . .	● Concept Development Teaching Strategy
● To develop skills of . . .	● Skill Development Teaching Strategy
● To develop awareness of values relative to . . .	● Values Awareness Teaching Strategy
● To develop inquiry strategies relative to . . .	● Inquiry Development Teaching Strategy
● To express ideas and discuss opinions and ideas relative to . . .	● Open-ended Discussion Teaching Strategy

To minimize the possibility of mismatching the teacher's goals for students and the teaching strategy utilized, in addition to the lesson flow, it is helpful to recognize some of the characteristic teacher and student roles of each of these teaching strategies. A list of characteristic student and teacher roles is also provided for each teaching strategy. While it is readily apparent that any lesson can be successfully implemented without all of the roles outlined, the roles do enable the reader to identify the commonalities and uniqueness of the teaching strategies discussed.

As each of the characteristic roles for the six teaching strategies is read, it should be noted that there are no teacher roles listed such as warm, friendly, humane, thoughtful, empathetic, and so on. This has not been an oversight. Rather, words such as these deal more with the nature of the affective lesson climate in which all of the roles listed are implemented. For example, one characteristic teacher role in a Concept Development lesson is to provide feedback — the means whereby the teacher lets the students know when they are "on-course" or "off-course" in relation to the concept being taught. This feedback can be given in a straightforward, impersonal way; it can be given in a way that tends to demean the students; or it can be given in a warm, friendly, humane, empathetic and thoughtful way.

The Information Acquisition Teaching Strategy

Some goals teachers have for their students may be classified as information acquisition. That is, the central emphasis of these lessons is on getting some information from the teacher, the health text, the district health curriculum guides, or other sources into the minds of students. Goals of many health education programs, for example, include giving students information about the major body parts and organs and their function, factors that characterize a healthy community, various sources of disease, differences between inherited and acquired characteristics, the names of various professions which promote and maintain health, definitions of health-related terms, factors that are believed to influence drug use and abuse, the function of different nutrients for the body, and so on.

The following is a sketch of the flow of a typical Information Acquisition Teaching Strategy.

Phase I: Introducing the Lesson

The information to be acquired by the students is previewed, including why they are to acquire that information and how it relates to preceding or following lessons.

Phase II: Implementing the Lesson

To achieve this kind of goal, the information is either presented to the students as the teacher shows or tells them the information, gives assigned readings in textbooks, magazines or pamphlets, shows a film, invites a guest speaker to the classroom, takes the class on a field trip, and so on. During the lesson, the teacher may also restate or recast the information as necessary for the students and respond to the students' requests for clarification.

Most frequently, the Information Acquisition Teaching Strategy tends to begin and end during the course of one lesson. That is, the information to be acquired by students is identified as the lesson goal. The lesson is then taught, and the students hopefully acquire that information as a result. There are exceptions to this generality, however. In an Information Acquisition lesson designed to inform the students about health services available in the community, for example, one teacher spent part of a lesson setting the stage for the topic by reviewing what a health service is. His students were then given a series of pamphlets about various health services available in the community and they were asked to read them. Then, for the next several days in the classroom, the teacher used a series of questions designed to get selected information about health services the students had read listed on a chart. The particular Information Acquisition lesson described took three lesson periods to implement.

Characteristic roles of the teacher during the introductory phase of an Information Acquisition lesson include:

• Presenting the lesson objective.
• Specifying the lesson structure, including:
  —how the students are to work,
  —the materials and facilities they'll use,
  —what they can expect of their teacher.

The student's roles during this phase include:

• Attending.
• Raising questions about the information to be acquired, the reason(s) they are to acquire the information or about the lesson structure.

Characteristic roles of the teacher during the implementation phase of the lesson include:

• Presenting the information or directing students to specified information.
• Acting to implement and maintain the lesson structure.
• Monitoring the student's responses to the presentation.
• Providing feedback, positive reinforcement and psychological support for the students as necessary.

The student's roles during this phase include:

• Working within the bounds of the lesson structure as outlined.
• Attending to the information presented.
• Sorting out relevant from irrelevant and "nice to know" from "must know" information.
• Recording relevant information as appropriate so it is available to them at a later time.
• Asking for clarification when they need help in understanding the information presented.

As an outgrowth of this teaching strategy, the students should be able to do such things as identify, distinguish, describe, recall, or retrace the specified information they have acquired.

The Concept Development Teaching Strategy

Some goals teachers have for their students may be classified as concept development. That is, the central emphasis of these lessons is to help the students develop their understanding of health concepts or generalizations. Many health education programs, for example, include concepts and/or generalizations such as: "Growing and developing follows a predictable sequence, yet is unique for each individual"; "There are reciprocal relationships involving man, disease and the environment"; "The family serves to perpetuate man and to fulfill certain health needs"; "Use of substances that modify mood and behavior arises from a variety of motivations"; "Food selection and eating patterns are determined by physical, social, mental, economic and cultural factors."[8]

The following is a sketch of the flow of a typical Concept Development Teaching Strategy.

Phase I: Introducing the Lesson

The concept or generalization to be developed is previewed, including why the students are to develop the concept. In addition, this lesson may be related to previous or following lessons as necessary.

Phase II: Implementing the Lesson

Through a discussion, group activity or individual work, the teacher involves the students in recalling, generating and processing data in order to build a generalization. While lessons intended only to develop a generalization are through at this point, Concept Development lessons continue as the teacher uses additional activities or questions and statements to stimulate the students' use of those intellectual processes on data or other concepts as necessary to build or assimilate the "new" concept. Certainly the concepts which result are directly influenced by on-course and off-course feedback, restatements and elaborations by the teacher or by the students' use of specially prepared materials intended to insure the development of the desired concept.

Finally, because concepts are to be used, students test their "new" concept as the teacher creates opportunities for them to use it to develop a model, explanation, prediction, hypothesis, make a judgment, formulate a course of action, or relate the "new" concept to a concept previously learned.

While the Information Acquisition Teaching Strategy usually takes the period of one lesson to accomplish the lesson objective, a Concept Development Teaching Strategy more frequently involves more than one lesson to implement. Depending on the complexity of the concept to be taught, a Concept Development Teaching Strategy could run over the course of several lessons. While a Concept Development lesson may include giving students certain information and getting the students to implement specified intellectual skills, the lesson success criteria center primarily on the consideration of the students ability to use the specified concept(s). Any information students acquire or intellectual skill they practice are not, therefore, the major concern of a Concept Development Teaching Strategy.

Characteristic roles of the teacher during the introductory phase of a Concept Development lesson include:

- Presenting the lesson objective.
- Specifying the lesson structure including:
  —how the students are to work,
  —the materials and facilities they will use,
  —what they can expect of their teacher.

The students' roles during this phase include:

- Attending.
- Raising questions about the concept, the reason(s) they are to learn the concept, or about the lesson structure.
- Proposing alternative ways of working within the bounds established by the teacher.

Characteristic roles of the teachers during the implementation phase of the lesson include:

- Initiating an activity, sequence of activities, or utilizing a series of concept-related questions or statements to facilitate concept development.
- Acting to implement and maintain the lesson structure.
- Monitoring student participation.
- Guiding students by cluing, cueing, summarizing, ...
- Providing feedback, positive reinforcement, and psychological support for the students as they work.

The students' roles during this phase include:

- Working within the bounds of the lesson structure as outlined.
- Participating in the activity(ies) and/or responding to the teacher's questions or statements as appropriate.

* Asking for clarification when they experience some confusion in what they are to do, how they are to do it, or when they have not understood the teacher or another student.

As an outgrowth of this teaching strategy, the students should be able to use the concept outside of the setting in which it was developed. For example, the teacher may create a situation in which the students are expected to use a given concept to develop an explanation for a phenomenon "new" to them, to formulate a course of action consistent with the concept, to use a concept to make a prediction consistent with the concept, to use the concept to make a judgment, to use the concept to develop a hypothesis, to build a model consistent with the concept, and so on.

The Skill Development Teaching Strategy

Some goals teachers have for their students may be classified as intellectual or psychomotor skill building. While to achieve this kind of goal, teachers may tell students about a skill they are to learn, point out how the skill may be useful to them, and describe or demonstrate the specific skill to be learned, the central emphasis of these lessons is on the students' attainment of the skill so they are able to use it when they choose to do so. Many health education programs, for example, include intellectual skills such as *analyzing* claims made for and against fluoridation, *summarizing* individual health problems that may result from poor dietary habits, *interpreting* data about smoking and the occurrence of disease, *translating* health data about over-the-counter medicines presented in graph form to narrative form, and psychomotor skills such as brushing teeth, *exercising* to increase cardiorespiratory efficiency and so on.

The following is a sketch of the flow of a typical Skill Development Teaching Strategy.

Phase I: Introducing the Lesson

The skill to be developed by the students is previewed, including why they are to develop the skill, how they will know when to use the skill and so on. In addition, this lesson may be related to previous or following lessons as necessary.

Phase II: Implementing the Lesson

To achieve this kind of goal, the skill to be developed is demonstrated for the students either by the teacher, through a film, through some reading material or study prints or other such material. Then the students are invited to go through the skill step-by-step with the teacher giving corrective feedback to them as they follow along. Following this beginning work, the students are then given the opportunity to practice the skill at increasing levels of difficulty, with the teacher monitoring their work, giving corrective feedback and psychological support and reteaching the students as needed.

Of course, there are instances in which the teacher may just begin the skill development by demonstrating the skill and then inviting the students to practice it. In this case, step-by-step help may be then given to individual students, or to the entire group, as necessary.

Whatever else happens as part of Skill Development lessons, students must have sufficient opportunities to both practice the desired skill and to get feedback on their performance if they are to achieve this kind of goal. Feedback may be given to the students directly by the teacher, it may be built into the materials through the inclusion of some sort of answer sheet, or the students may be given some criteria they can use to determine if they were right or wrong for themselves. Regardless of which of these approaches is used, the more immediate and precise the feedback, the more positive its effect on the student's learning.

Like the Concept Development Teaching Strategy, a Skill Development Teaching Strategy may include giving students certain information. In this case, the information provided would probably be in relation to the skill to be learned. It is conceivable also that the teacher might review certain concepts the student may have learned at an earlier date that the student will need during the Skill Development lesson. Regardless of the information given and concepts reviewed, however, the lesson success criterion centers primarily on developing the student's ability to use the specified intellectual or psychomotor skill(s) effectively.

Because most Skill Development lessons proceed through a sequence of informing students about what the skill is and what people can do with it, taking students through the implementation of the skill and giving them time to practice the skill, the Skill Development Teaching Strategy usually runs for the period of more than one lesson. Surely, however, there are some Skill Development objectives that may be accomplished during the period of one lesson.

Characteristic roles of the teacher during the introductory phase of a Skill Development lesson include:

* Outlining the lesson objective.
* Specifying the lesson structure including:
  —how the students are to work to develop the skill,
  —the materials and facilities they'll use,
  —what the students can expect of their teacher.

The students' roles during this phase include:

* Attending.
* Raising questions about the skill, the reason(s) they are to learn the skill or about the lesson structure.
* Proposing alternative ways of working.

Characteristic roles of the teacher during the implementation phase of the lesson include:

* Introducing the skill by describing and/or demonstrating it as appropriate.
* Initiating a practice/skill development activity.
* Acting to implement and maintain the lesson structure.
* Monitoring student participation to diagnose where students experience difficulty and provide assistance as necessary.
* Providing feedback, positive reinforcement, and psychological support for the students as they work.

The students' roles during this phase include:

* Attending to information about the skill.
* Participating in the Skill Development activity(ies).
* Asking for clarification when they experience some confusion in what they are to do or how they are to do it.
* Asking for help when they experience some demands beyond their present capabilities.

As an outgrowth of this teaching strategy, the students should be able to perform the intellectual skills or psychomotor skills taught.

The Values Awareness Teaching Strategy

Some goals teachers have for their students may be classified as awareness. That is, the central emphasis of these lessons is both on helping students become aware of their values in relation to specified topics and on developing their ability to explicate their values on their own. Many health education programs, for example, seek to help students become aware of their values about issues like fluoridation, family planning, euthanasia, medicare, government control of medicines, drug advertising, fad foods, premarital sex, venereal diseases, and so on.

The following is a sketch of the flow of a typical Values Awareness Teaching Strategy.

Phase I: Introducing the Lesson

The teacher may initiate an activity or an introductory discussion either to surface a discussion topic of interest to the students or to set the stage for a topic predetermined by the teacher. This introductory discussion or stage setting concludes with the identification of the topic or question for the discussion.

Phase II: Implementing the Lesson

To achieve this kind of goal, the teacher involves the students in a values-loaded discussion or activity that centers on inviting the students to use their values by making a value judgment or recommending a course of action. As the students do so, the teacher works to help the students gain insight into some of the values which underlie those value judgments or courses of action. During the discussion, the teacher also maintains the lesson structure.

Near the close of the lesson, the teacher occasionally initiates a lesson Process Dialogue that is intended to invite the students to reflect on what they did during the discussion and how they felt about the lesson in general.

Depending on how long the teacher takes to set the stage for the topic and the way the students respond to the discussion question, there may be occasions in which the Values Awareness Teaching Strategy may run over the course of several Values Awareness lessons. More frequently, however, since most lessons are implemented through a discussion format, the Values Awareness Teaching Strategy occurs within the period of one lesson.

Characteristic roles of the teacher during the introductory phase of a Values Awareness Teaching Strategy include:

* Outlining the lesson objective.
* Specifying the lesson structure including:
  —how students are to work in the lesson,
  —the materials and facilities they will use,
  —what the students can expect of their teacher.

The student's roles during this phase include:

* Attending.
* Raising questions about the lesson topic, the reason(s) why they are to discuss that topic or about the lesson structure.
* Proposing alternative ways of working.

Characteristic roles of the teacher during the implementation phase of the lesson include:

* Initiating the lesson.
* Acting to implement the lesson structure.
* Utilizing specified teacher interventions to help students become aware of the various processes they utilize, consider the conditions relative to their recommendations and become aware of their values.
* Utilizing specified diagnostic teacher behaviors intended to help the teacher diagnose student growth.
* Conducting a post-process dialogue to invite the students to report on their ways of working, etc.

The students' roles during this phase include:

* Attending.
* Participating in the lesson by reporting value judgments, courses of action, making predictions, reporting data, reporting values, generating data and so on.
* Working within the bounds of the lesson structure as outlined.
* Asking for clarification by the teacher or other students when they do not understand what was said and they want to.

As an outgrowth of this teaching strategy, the students should be able to report their values in relation to specified subjects suitable for classroom discussion, relate an individual's or group's values to the actions, decisions, or judgments they make, and so on.

The Inquiry Development Teaching Strategy

Some goals teachers have for their students may be classified as inquiry strategy development. That is, the central emphasis of these

lessons is both on the development of the students' repertoire of
problem solving strategies and their positive self-concept as effective
problem solvers. To achieve this goal many health education
programs, for example, use problems such as, "Despite the known
harmful effects of smoking and in the fact of repeated warnings by the
Surgeon General, why is it that close to 50 percent of all people in the
United States 17 years of age and older smoke cigarettes?" "Why is it
that the incidence of smallpox has decreased dramatically during the
last four years?" "Why is the incidence of heart disease greater in the
United States than it is in Japan?"

The following is a sketch of the flow of a typical Inquiry
Development Teaching Strategy.

Phase I: Introducing the Lesson

The teacher may use a demonstration, photographs, charts, a
discussion, etc, to set the stage for the inquiry problem. This
may be preceded with or followed by a pre-Process Dialogue
intended to invite the students to consider various inquiry
strategies they will use to build and/or test their theories as
they work to solve the problem.

Phase II: Implementing the Lesson

Once the students are informed of the health-related inquiry
problem, the teacher makes it possible for the students to
work on the problem in their own way and at their own pace.
Depending on the specific problem at hand and the way the
students prefer to work, they may work as individuals, work
in groups, or work as a total class. During their work time,
the teacher maintains the lesson structure and uses specific
teaching behaviors to facilitate the students' growth toward
the lesson goals.

The students' work on the problem concludes as they are
invited to participate in a Post-Process Dialogue. At this time,
they are invited to reflect on their work — the processes and
strategies they used to build and test their theories and how
well those processes and strategies they used helped them
work toward an effective solution for the problem.

Depending on the way the teacher sets the stage for the inquiry
problem, the way the students are to generate data, how involved the
problem is, how interested the students are in the problem, and how
much experience the students have had with inquiry, an Inquiry

Teaching Strategy may range from one class period to a problem the students may work on over a semester. More frequently, however, an Inquiry Teaching Strategy may range from two to five inquiry lessons.

Characteristic roles of the teacher during the introductory phase of an Inquiry lesson include:

- Specifying the inquiry problem the students are to work on.
- Specifying the lesson structure including:
  —how the students are to work,
  —the materials and facilities they will use,
  —what the students can expect of their teacher.

The students' roles during this phase include:

- Attending.
- Raising questions about the problem, why they are to have an Inquiry lesson or about the lesson structure.
- Proposing alternative ways of working.
- Participating in the pre-process dialogue by naming or describing inquiry processes and strategies useful in working on the problem.

Characteristic roles of the teacher during the implementation phase of the lesson include:

- Initiating the lesson.
- Acting to implement and maintain the lesson structure.
- Making data available to the students as they request it.
- Providing process help to the students appropriate to their level of inquiry development.
- Using diagnostic teaching behaviors to assess student growth.
- Conducting a post-process dialogue.

Characteristic students' roles during this phase include:

- Attending.
- Using a range of inquiry processes and strategies while working to solve the problem.
- Identifying other inquiry problems.
- Working within the bounds of the lesson structure as outlined.
- Participating in the post-process dialogue by reporting the effectiveness of the various inquiry processes and strategies used.
- Asking for clarification by the teacher or other students when they do not understand what was said — and they want to.

As an outgrowth of this teaching strategy, the students should be able to label the various inquiry processes they or others use, prescribe and utilize a range of theory-building and theory-testing strategies, report or describe the various strategies they use, etc.

The Open-Ended Discussion Teaching Strategy

Some goals teachers have for their students may be classified as interpersonal communication. That is, the central emphasis of these lessons is on developing the students' abilities to express and discuss opinions and ideas related to a range of topics. To do so means the students must first give some thought to how they feel about the topic. As far as the students are concerned, one of the major outcomes is to enable the students to find out where they are and where their friends are in their thinking at the time.

The following is a sketch of the flow of a typical Open-Ended Discussion Teaching Strategy.

Phase I: Introducing the Lesson

The teacher may initiate an activity or an introductory discussion either to surface a discussion topic of interest to the students or to set the stage for a predetermined discussion topic by the teacher. This introductory discussion or stage setting concludes with the identification of the topic or question for the discussion.

Phase II: Implementing the Lesson

To achieve this type of goal, the teacher makes it possible for the students to participate in small and/or large group discussions to express their attitudes, opinions, value judgments, and ideas in a responsible and thoughtful way. The discussion centers on student/student dialogue. During the lesson, the teacher's major task is to maintain the lesson structure.

Depending on how the teacher sets the stage for the topic and the way the students respond to the discussion question, there may be occasions in which the Open-Ended Discussion Teaching Strategy may run over the course of several discussion lessons. More frequently, however, the Open-Ended Discussion will begin and end within the period of one lesson.

Characteristic roles of the teacher during the introductory phase of an Open-Ended Discussion include:
- Outlining the lesson objective.
- Specifying the lesson structure including:
  —how the students are to work,
  —what they can expect of their teacher.

The students' roles during the lesson include:

- Attending.
- Raising questions about the discussion topic, the reason(s) they are to discuss that topic or about the lesson structure.
- Proposing alternative ways of working.

Characteristic roles of the teacher during the implementation phase of the lesson include:

- Initiating the discussion.
- Acting to implement and maintain the lesson structure.

The students' roles during this phase include:

- Attending.
- Participating in the discussion by sharing ideas, opinions, feelings, seeking data, reporting data, seeking clarification, making value judgments, etc.
- Working within the bounds of the lesson structure as outlined.
- Asking for clarification by the teacher or other students when they do not understand what was said and they want to.

As an outgrowth of this teaching strategy, students should be willing and able to report their own position on a given topic or issue, get feedback from their peers, learn the position of others in their class about that issue or topic, become more effective in interacting with others, etc.

Relationships Among the Different Teaching Strategies

In this discussion about teaching strategies, each of the six have been presented as a specific, discrete way of working in the classroom. And each is. However, when we turn our attention to day-to-day teaching in the classroom, we find that students' learning is a product of the sequence of teaching strategies they experience rather than individual teaching strategies used in isolation from each other. This ability to establish relationships among certain teaching strategies adds another element to the complexities, and the power of teaching.

One kind of relationship among teaching strategies is a diagnostic one. That is, the act of using one teaching strategy toward a specified objective may give the teacher diagnostic information about what the students know or do not know, their level of development of certain skills, concepts they lack or misconcepts they hold, or their ability to discuss health-related topics. Other teaching strategies may then be designed or redesigned to meet these identified student needs. For example, during a Values Awareness discussion that centered on the question, "How do you feel about rising welfare costs?" the teacher may learn about misconcepts the students hold about the health practices of a particular ethnic group. A Skill Development lesson which centers on drawing inferences from data might then be developed and used with the students so they work with valid data about the ethnic group in question. The teacher can, therefore, develop the students' skill in graphing data while at the same time providing the data necessary to reshape their misconcepts. Or, the misconcepts students hold may be dealt with through an Information Acquisition Teaching Strategy designed to get the accurate information about the specific ethnic group to the students.

A second kind of relationship among teaching strategies is what we call "by-product learning." By "by-product learning," we mean learning that takes place in addition to the learning identified as the major lesson objective. For example, one intellectual skill for students to develop in the area of health education is the ability to interpret and summarize data which is presented in graph or chart form. Since in one instance a class was involved in a unit of study centered on the prevention of diseases or disorders, the teacher invited students to build bar graphs about the occurrence of smallpox over the last 20 years in countries where vaccination is used. They then compared these data to other graphs they made about the occurrence of smallpox over the last 20 years in those countries where vaccination is not used. Thus, while the major objective of this illustrative skill lesson was to develop the student's ability to interpret and summarize data presented in graph form, the data they worked with was also intended to reinforce the "prevention of diseases and disorders" information they learned in a prior lesson when the Information Acquisition Teaching Strategy was utilized.

This example of a "by-product learning" relationship among teaching strategies is true of teaching strategies in addition to Skill Development and Information Acquisition. With the Concept Development Teaching Strategy, for example, students process information to build the desired concept. While the major lesson objective is development of that concept, the teaching strategy may be designed so the students use certain intellectual skills learned during earlier Skill Development lessons such as drawing inferences from data, validating data, summarizing data, and so on. The Concept Development lesson, therefore, gave students additional practice in using such intellectual skills.

A third and more usual kind of relationship among teaching strategies is the orchestration of a sequence of different teaching strategies around a given concept or body of content to be developed. Consider the concept of immunization, for example. A unit of study may be initiated with an Information Acquisition Teaching Strategy designed to inform students about various kinds of immunizations presently available in the community. A Concept Development Teaching Strategy may be used to develop the students' concept about immunization, how it was developed, what happens in the body, etc. Predictions can be formulated as students work with data about immunization in relation to the occurrence of specified diseases such as influenza, smallpox, and diphtheria. An Open-Ended Discussion Teaching Strategy may be utilized to make it possible for students to discuss how they feel about getting immunizations. Finally, a topic such as, "How do you feel about people who don't take action to prevent disease for their children through immunization?" may be used as the topic for a Values Awareness Teaching Strategy in order to help the students become aware of their own values in relation to this issue. Used in this way, each of these teaching strategies supports the learning of the other. Seen as a whole, the range of teaching strategies offer the students a wide array of interrelated and mutually supportive learning experiences in relation to the subject matter to be taught to students.

The Six Teaching Strategies — Some Fundamental Differences

It is interesting to note that when the Six Teaching Strategies discussed earlier are compared, they fall into two groups. One group includes the Information Acquisition, Concept Development, and Skill Development Teaching Strategies. These teaching strategies center on the development of base line learning. Base line learning refers to that information and those concepts and skills deemed important in Health Education. The second group includes the Values Awareness, Inquiry, and Open-Ended Discussion Teaching Strategies. The emphasis of these teaching strategies is on the development of personal meaning. Personal meaning refers to the internalization of information, concepts and skills that take place as the students utilize the information, concepts and skills in (1) discussing health issues, (2) solving health problems suitable for use in the classroom, and (3) making health related decisions. In doing so, the students not only gain new insights as a result of their participation, but they also recognize how much more powerful they are because of the information, concepts, and skills they were able to bring to bear on their work.

In comparing these two groups of teaching strategies further, another difference between them becomes apparent. The nature of the goals for the base line learning teaching strategies — Information Acquisition, Concept Development, and Skill Development — are such that it is necessary for the teacher to provide on-course/off-course feedback for the students during the lesson in relation to the lesson content to let them know how they are doing. For example: *Right on, Swami; That's not what I had in mind, Vigero;* or, *You certainly did that very well, Jamie.*

The use of off-course feedback frequently creates the need for the teacher to provide psychological support. In doing so, the teacher communicates his or her support of and confidence in the student regardless of an incorrect answer given. A basic function of psychological support is to reinforce the student's participation in the lesson even though what the student may have contributed was incorrect or missed the point. For example: *Keep it up Cheryl, you'll get it.*

The nature of the goals for the personal meaning teaching strategies — Values Awareness, Inquiry Development, and Open-Ended Discussion — are such that for these teaching strategies to become effective, students must develop confidence in their ability to decide if they are right or wrong for themselves. This comes about most effectively when the teacher structures the lesson so students are responsible to generate their own on-course/off-course feedback about their work. As a result, they develop rational ways to decide for themselves. They come to find their own positive reinforcement in a job well done rather in being dependent on someone else making judgments about their work for them. They come to view difficulties they experience as they work as a positive learning experience which leads to personal growth rather than respond to it as a negative experience.

There are also other kinds of differences between the base line learning teaching strategies and the personal meaning teaching strategies. In Information Acquisition, Concept Development, and Skill Development Teaching Strategies, the teacher carries the responsibility for the lesson momentum. In Values Awareness, Inquiry, and Open-Ended Discussion Teaching Strategies, the students carry the responsibility for the lesson momentum.

Finally, the base line learning teaching strategies tend to be convergent in character for the students while the personalized meaning teaching strategies tend to be more divergent in character for them. That is, in base line learning teaching strategies, the lesson converges on the information the students are to acquire, the skills they are to develop, or the concepts they are to learn. On the other hand, personalized meaning teaching strategies are successful to the degree that students develop their own feelings, attitudes, or abilities.

Teaching Strategies — Some Afterthoughts

Most Teaching Strategies are Mutually Exclusive

In general, the six teaching strategies outlined are mutually exclusive. This is the case because each teaching strategy has some unique characteristic roles for the teacher and the students. For example, corrective feedback by the teacher is such a characteristic of a Skill Development Teaching Strategy. A critical characteristic of the Inquiry Teaching Strategy is that students generate their own feedback about their work. Thus, if the teacher gives corrective feedback to students during an Inquiry lesson, that action would interfere with the Inquiry goals. On the other hand, if the teacher were not to give corrective feedback to students during a Skill Development lesson, it is questionable whether the Skill Development goals would be accomplished.

Teaching Without Learning

Some kinds of desired learning in the public schools may appear to take place without "teaching." Classroom utilization of programmed instructional materials, learning centers, contract learning packages, workbooks, films and other mediated instructional materials illustrate this point. During these kinds of lessons, the teacher functions mainly in a management role. This is not learning without teaching. It is just that in these instances, the "teacher" is the person who developed the classroom materials. The developer/teacher's influence is felt through the questions, judgments, data, and ideas built into the educational material produced. It is as though the teacher role is being filled by a teacher "in absentia."

Teaching vs Learning

Frequently, discussion presentations or articles about instruction dichotomize teaching and learning. That is, one kind of instruction may be emphasized which stresses learning (which is good) as compared to some other kind of instruction that emphasizes teaching (which is bad). In our view, this dichotomy leads to the position that learning can take place without teaching, and more significantly, that good teaching can and indeed does take place without learning!! While it is true that learning does occur without teaching, it is our belief that the central thrust of public education is toward those kinds of learnings that occur as a result of teaching — learning we do not want to let go to chance. Teaching and learning must, therefore, be viewed not as bad and good aspects of instruction respectively, but rather as interdependent components. A measure of the effectiveness of teaching is the accomplishment of the desired learning.

Classroom Organizational Practices are not Teaching Strategies

The reader may recall that none of the teaching strategies outlined in these materials carry the label *Individualized Instruction, Small Group Instruction,* or *Nongraded Instruction,* or... It is not because there is an objective to what these labels stand for, rather Individualized Instruction, Small Group Instruction, Nongraded...are viewed as ways of organizing students for instruction. While such classroom organizational patterns are an important element of the effective implementation of any teaching strategy, an organizational pattern in and of itself is not a teaching strategy. For example, as an organizational pattern, Individualized Instruction may be used for either Information Acquisition, Concept Development, or Skill Development goals. The way a classroom is organized is, therefore, only one element of any teaching strategy.

7

Selecting and Building the Appropriate Teaching Strategy: A Three-Step Process

One critical task of the health educator is to select the appropriate teaching strategy for the goal(s) sought for students at the time.

Six teaching strategies; which is best? Such is the teacher's dilemma. Certainly there are instances in which a teacher deals with only one of the goals for his students, so only one kind of teaching strategy is probably used in his or her classroom. A comprehensive program in health education, however, should deal with all six of the teacher's goals for students outlined. Six teaching strategies; which is best? It all depends on the goal sought at the time.

What follows are three steps that move from the identification or selection of the lesson objective to building of the lesson. Certainly the act of designing and implementing a teaching strategy to achieve a specified objective for students requires more than just being able to state these three steps. It is a demanding, difficult, complex, and creative task. No one ever said that good teaching was easy. Mastery of a network of teaching skills as well as a depth of knowledge about the subject matter are necessary if these three steps are to be implemented effectively. The act of presenting this three-step process is not intended to structure teaching so as to inhibit a teacher's creativity and experimentation. Rather, the process is useful because it provides a framework that serves to stimulate a teacher's creative efforts. Knowing the nature of the teaching strategy to be created makes the job somewhat more productive.

Step I:
Identifying the Lesson Objective(s)

Since the fundamental purpose of a teaching strategy is to facilitate student achievement of specific lesson objective(s), the selection of the most appropriate teaching strategy begins after a lesson objective is identified. Some teachers begin by formulating objectives for the class based on what they perceive to be the health needs of their students. Certainly this does not mean that all of the objectives for a health education class or unit of study must be crystalized at the beginning of the school year. They may be designed for a unit of study, or even on a day-to-day basis. On the other hand, many teachers have a set of objectives for health education already developed or made available by their school district. In this case, teachers have only to choose or modify objectives as appropriate for their class. It is only a question of which objectives are most relevant for their students. In some instances, a pretest may be used. In some instances, objectives may be chosen on a basis of professional judgment — what the teacher knows of his or her students and the subject matter related to health education. In any case, the message is clear. The building of a teaching strategy begins with the identification of what the students are to learn.

Step II:
Selecting the Appropriate Teaching Strategy

Having decided what the students are to learn, the next question is, what teaching strategy will be used to facilitate that learning? Because each of the goals outlined requires a different teaching strategy and each teaching strategy carries some unique student and teacher roles, problems arise when teachers inadvertently mismatch a lesson goal and teaching strategy. For example, Concept Development lessons frequently fail in the classroom because teachers use an Information Acquisition Teaching Strategy to try to do the job. While the Information Acquisition Teaching Strategy does involve students in recalling information, this teaching strategy does not engage students in processing information. However, Concept Development is dependent on the students' utilization of intellectual processes such as analyzing and synthesizing information related to the given concept. Thus, Concept Development seldom happens as a predictable outgrowth of using the Information Acquisition Teaching Strategy except by chance. And the same is true of the other teaching strategies as well. It is critical, therefore, that the teacher deliberately match the lesson goal with the appropriate teaching strategy.

The task of selecting the appropriate teaching strategy begins as the teacher relates a given lesson objective to one of the six general goals for students. It involves classifying the objective in student terms as either to: (1) acquire information, (2) develop a specified concept, (3) develop a specified skill, (4) become aware of individual values, (5) develop inquiry strategies, or (6) express and discuss opinions and ideas.

One way to classify an objective is to consider the student behavior called for. If the student is to demonstrate acquisition of specific information by completing a multiple choice test, for example, the objective would seem to be related to the Information Acquisition goal. If the student is to demonstrate understanding of a specified concept by using it outside of the context in which it was learned to formulate a prediction, course of action, a judgment, build an explanation, develop a hypotheses, or build a model based on the concept, that objective would seem to be related to the Concept Development goal. If the student is to demonstrate the ability to perform a specific psychomotor or intellectual skill, that objective would seem to be related to the Skill Development goal. If the student is to demonstrate he or she has developed a theory-testing strategy useful in dealing effectively with a given health-related problem by prescribing, implementing and evaluating that strategy, that objective would seem to be related to the Inquiry Strategies goal. Finally, if the student is to demonstrate his or her ability and willingness to participate as a member of a group exploring a given health issue by reporting opinions or ideas, reporting or generating data, or taking action to understand the ideas of others in a thoughtful and responsible way, that objective would seem to be related to the Expression and Discussion of Opinions and Ideas goal.

As a result of trying to classify a lesson objective as one of the six goals for instruction, the teacher may find that either the objective is difficult to classify or that the resulting goal or teaching strategy just does not "feel right."

This probably is an indication that the objective may have to be revised or rewritten because it does not communicate exactly what you feel it should; it does not represent the learning you feel is important for your students; or, this kind of analysis may reveal that a particular "objective" is actually a learning activity.

An activity outlines a learning experience for the students — what they are to do during the lesson. An activity specifies one way of doing something — a specific task in which the students are to participate. The following is an illustration of an activity.

Given the necessary ingredients, recipe, and utensils, the students will prepare pancakes.

While the foregoing may look like an objective, it does not indicate what the students are to learn as they participate in the activity outlined. An objective specifies the purpose or learning outcome of instruction and is frequently, though not always, stated in some measurable terms. The following is an illustration of what an objective for the preceding activity might look like.

The students will be able to use a simple recipe to prepare a food. The food prepared will be consistent with the recipe provided.

While there is only one way of implementing an activity, an objective may be achieved through different activities. It is important to note that both objectives and activities are needed for instruction. If after an analysis an "objective" turns out to be an activity the teacher feels is important for the students, the question then is, "What is it the students are to learn as they participate in the activity?" Stated another way the question is, *"What is/are the lesson objectives?"*

With the objective classified as one of the six goals for instruction, the teaching strategy most appropriate to facilitate the achievement of that objective is evident (Figure 8).

FIGURE 8

Teacher's Goals for Students	Related Teaching Strategies
● To acquire information about . . .	● Information Acquisition Teaching Strategy
● To develop concepts about . . .	● Concept Development Teaching Strategy
● To develop skills of . . .	● Skill Development Teaching Strategy
● To develop awareness of values relative to . . .	● Values Awareness Teaching Strategy
● To develop inquiry strategies relative to . . .	● Inquiry Development Teaching Strategy
● To express ideas and discuss opinions and ideas relative to . . .	● Open-ended Discussion Teaching Strategy

Step III:
Building the Teaching Strategy

Critical to the success of any lesson is the successful implementation of the characteristic student and teacher roles. The various roles outlined in the description of each teaching strategy, therefore, serve as a guide in building a lesson to ensure an internal consistency between what the students and teachers do and the lesson objective.

With the teaching strategy identified, the lesson flow and student

FIGURE 9

LESSON OBJECTIVE: Given a balanced meal in menu or picture form, the student will be able to analyze the meal for range of nutrients found in the foods and report those observations orally or in written form.

Student Roles	and	Related Student Activities
Attend to information about the skill.		Listen and observe.
Participate in skill development activity.		Analyze menus from local restaurants and report observations about the range of nutrients found in the meals.

Teacher Roles	and	Related Teaching Techniques and Behaviors
Introduce skills.		Use overhead projector to describe and demonstrate analysis of a meal for range and amount of nutrients.
Initiate practice activity.		Use overhead projector to inform students about working areas and their roles during the lesson practice activity.
Monitor student participation to diagnose where students experience difficulty and provide assistance as necessary.		Observe students at work.
Provide feedback.		Let students know how they are doing verbally while they work or use specially prepared cassette tapes for individual feedback.

and teacher roles are identified. What remains to be done is to: (1) decide on suitable activities for students that make it possible for them to implement their roles in the lesson and master the lesson objective(s), (2) identify teaching techniques and teaching behaviors through which the teacher roles are implemented, and (3) identify the specified materials needed and the classroom organizational pattern most appropriate.

To illustrate this process, Figure 9 shows some notes a teacher has made in doing some preliminary planning for a Skill Development lesson. While not all teachers find it necessary to write their ideas down in this way, we have used this approach as a way to share the teacher's thinking with the reader.

As Figure 9 shows, the lesson begins to take shape. With the lesson objective identified, the appropriate teaching strategy was selected. In view of the characteristic student and teacher roles, specific activities were created or identified. Finally, specific materials were selected and the lesson is about ready to go. What remains to be done for the illustrative lesson on nutrients outlined earlier is to make arrangements to get the needed copies of menus from local restaurants, select the pictures of the meals from the National Dairy Council materials, make arrangements for an overhead projector for the classroom, prepare an analysis of the various meals to test out the task the students will do, identify the various student working areas and give some thought to their roles.

In summary, there is nothing special, unique, or mystical about selecting and implementing a teaching strategy. It is just one way of being a responsible professional who gives some deliberate thought to what it is the students are to learn, what they will do to learn it and what the teacher will do to facilitate that learning. It is called humane teaching. The process begins with the identification of the lesson goals and concludes when the teaching strategy has been implemented with students in the classroom.

8

The Values Awareness
Teaching Strategy —
An Overview

*Students develop a concept of value as
they come to understand themselves.
Then, they use that concept as a way to
understand the world around them.*

While developing students' knowledge of societal values is an
expected outcome of schooling, by no means is it enough. Parents
want the schools to do more than inform students about societal values alone. They also want their children to learn how to respond
effectively to the kinds of value-laden problems they will encounter in
their daily lives. Fundamental to the students' knowledge of societal
values and their ability to respond effectively to problems in the arena
of values are an operational concept of value and an awareness of
their own values. Developing an operational concept of values and the
student's ability to explicate their own values are primary goals of the
Values Awareness Teaching Strategy.

Values awareness lessons do not just happen in the classroom
because the students read a new textbook or because they participate
in some group activities. Values awareness is a complex, demanding,
and dynamic process which unfolds when the teacher creates a
classroom climate that fosters thoughtful and responsible interaction
among the students about topics appropriate for the classroom.

But values awareness takes more than an effective classroom
climate. In addition, the teacher must also know what interventions to
use that will help students move toward the goals of values awareness
lessons. Good intentions are not enough. The professional health
educator needs both relevant knowledge about values and what can be
done to facilitate values awareness, and the related skills necessary to
implement that knowledge effectively in the classroom.

The Flow of a Typical Values Awareness Lesson

In general, most values awareness lessons move through two distinct phases: Introducing the Lesson and Implementing the Lesson. To introduce a Values Awareness lesson the teacher must either state or surface the lesson topic and also establish the way of working — the lesson structure. The stage may be set for a lesson topic by engaging the students in a brief discussion about a transparency, picture, or slide, reading an appropriate short story aloud to the students or letting them read it silently by themselves; viewing an appropriate open-ended discussion starter film or filmstrip; re-capping a recent or current controversial school, community, national or world event; or, participating in a values clarification, simulation, or human relations activity.

With the stage set, the lesson topic is usually presented in a form of a discussion question. For a values awareness lesson, the most effective discussion questions are based on either of the following illustrative stems: *How do you feel about...?* or *What should be done about...?* Questions such as these invite students to make value judgments or suggest courses of action. To do either, people use their values. When students have done so, it is possible for the teacher to help them surface the values which underlie their judgments or the actions they have proposed. And that's what values awareness is all about.

Most frequently the values awareness lesson discussion question is presented to the group by the teacher. There are instances, however, in which the teacher designs the introductory phase of the lesson so the students suggest a topic or select one they would like to discuss from a list prepared by the teacher. Once the lesson topic has been adequately introduced and the students informed of how they are to work, the lesson moves into the Implementation Phase. Working either as a total class or in groups, the teacher implements the lesson by inviting the students to respond to the discussion question. As they do so, the teacher uses specific teaching behaviors through which: (1) the climate and integrity of the lesson is implemented (the lesson structure); (2) the student's growth toward values awareness goal is facilitated; and (3) the student's growth may be diagnosed.

The discussion is concluded as the teacher initiates the Post-Process Dialogue. This dialogue is a kind of debriefing session in which the students are invited to comment on such issues as what went on during the lesson, how they felt about their participation in the discussion, and so on. In essence, this part of the lesson is intended to help students reflect on their experience from both an intellectual and affective vantage point.

A Glimpse of a Values Awareness Lesson

To explore the flow of a Values Awareness Teaching Strategy further, it is helpful to review an illustrative lesson. In so doing it is possible to highlight those teaching behaviors useful in working toward values awareness lesson goals. It is also possible to get some feeling for the relationship between the students and their teacher. While the topic of the discussion in this illustrative lesson is more appropriate for junior and senior high school students in a health education class, the lesson climate and the teaching behaviors utilized are the same regardless of the age of the students or the subject matter.

Introducing the Lesson

Ms. Pollock's class was involved in a unit of study in the area of diseases and disorders. Up to this time the students had studied primarily about leading communicable diseases. In so doing they gained information about various kinds of communicable diseases and learned of ways that each disease they studied may be transmitted.

Ms. Pollock had also spent several lessons on developing the students' concept of immunity including what it is, how people become immune, and so on. In addition, some lessons were directed to helping the students learn to read and interpret data provided in selected charts and graphs as a way to determine the present and past occurrence of the diseases being studied.

One of the diseases studied that caught the students' attention because people do not develop an immunity to it, because of its prevalence, and because of the social stigma attached to it, was gonorrhea. In view of their interest, Ms. Pollock saw this as an opportunity to use gonorrhea as a topic which would help students become aware of their values about social responsibility in relation to communicable diseases.

To set the stage for the discussion, Ms. Pollock first made some general comments to the class about how they would work.

MS. POLLOCK: *What I would like to do is to invite you to think about a particular issue. I'm going to present this issue to you*

*in the form of a transparency. As we work I want you to feel
that you can share what you think should happen, or ought to
happen. I want you to feel comfortable in discussing the
situation as you see it.*

*You can share your own opinion about it or you can agree
or disagree with other people's ideas or opinions. If you want
some information, you can ask me and I'll try to give you the
information you want, if I have it. Also, let's have one person
talk at a time so we can hear what each person has to say.*

*I'm not going to call on anyone during the discussion. If
you have something you want to say, it's up to you to make
your comment. Raise your hand or just speak out if there's a
moment of silence. Also, I'm not going to act as an amplifier for
the group. If someone speaks and you can't hear or if you
couldn't understand what they were saying, it will be up to you
to let them know.*

*And I'm not going to make any judgments about anyone's
comments by saying things like, "Good idea" or "You're right,"
and so on.*

Then Ms. Pollock put a transparency she had adapted from the
School Health Education Study Materials† onto the overhead
projector. A reproduction of the transparency she used is shown in
Figure 10.

Ms. Pollock then invited the students to comment about what they
felt was happening in the transparency.

MS. POLLOCK: *Okay, let's begin. Can you tell me what's going
on here; what do you see happening?*

JOE: *Well, that guy got kind of busted for gonorrhea and he's
wondering what he should do about it.*

MS. POLLOCK: *Okay.*

ED: *Well, I don't think he's being busted. They just discovered
that he had it, and I bet he's trying to decide what to do about
it.*

MS. POLLOCK: *Then you're saying that he's just found out that
he has it and he's trying to figure out what he should do?*

ED: *Yes.*

---

†*Russell, RD: Illustrating How The Health Status of Any Family Member May Affect
Living Patterns of The Family Group. Visual Packet No. 4361, School Health Education
Study, St. Paul: 3M Company 1967. Visual T.*

JIM: *He's probably also afraid that his friends will find out that he has it and what might happen to him.*

MS. POLLOCK: *All right. It's kind of the way it seems, would you agree?*

STUDENTS: Several students nod in apparent agreement.

Okay, then. Here's the situation. Gerald is down at the Midtown Clinic and the doctor is telling him, "You've got gonorrhea."

FIGURE 10

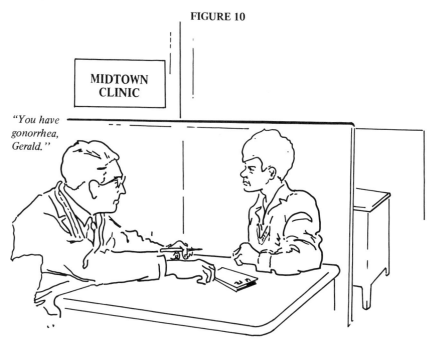

"You have
gonorrhea,
Gerald."

MIDTOWN
CLINIC

This brief discussion about the transparency assured that all of the students would interpret the transparency in the same way. The students' comments also set the stage for the teacher to pose the focus setting question, which she wrote along the bottom of the transparency as she spoke.

MS. POLLOCK: *Here's a question I'd like to invite you to respond to; "What do you think Gerald should do?"*

At this point the introductory phase of the lesson was complete. The teacher used a transparency on an overhead projector to set the stage for the discussion question she was to introduce. She also had set the lesson structure by informing the students about how they were to work. Of course, if the students had participated in several such discussions prior to this one, Ms. Pollock may have only commented that they would work as they had before. In this case, however, she chose to be more detailed in structuring for the lesson. Finally, the discussion question was presented to the group.

Implementing the Lesson

Having concluded the introductory phase of the lesson, Ms. Pollock used nonverbal communication to reinforce the lesson structure as she waited silently for them to respond to the discussion topic. After a few seconds of silence, one of the students spoke. The implementation phase of the lesson began.

JIM: *I'm wondering if the doctor is going to tell his mom and dad.*

MS. POLLOCK: *Are you asking me if the doctor has to tell his parents?*

JIM: *Yeah, if he has to tell them.*

MS. POLLOCK: *No. According to the California law right now, the doctor does not have to report to the parents of a minor when he or she has a venereal disease — syphilis or gonorrhea.*

JIM: *Then I think that Gerald guy should get the treatment. Right away!*

MS. POLLOCK: *Okay.*

ALETA: *But that's not all. He should also tell the girl he was with. She ought to know about it too.*

JAN: *I agree. She could have it and not know it and that could mess her up, but good.*

JACK: *Right. She could have given it to him or he might have given it to her.*

MS. POLLACK: *I see.*

DAPHNE: *Just think of all the girls Gerald could infect if he doesn't get treated, and...*

STUDENTS: Several students in the group laugh and begin commenting privately to each other about Daphne's comment.

MS. POLLOCK: *Wait a minute people, let's give Daphne a chance to finish what she has to say.*

DAPHNE: *Well I just wanted to say that it can give him lots of other trouble too.*

MS. POLLOCK: *What do you mean by other trouble, Daphne?*

DAPHNE: *It will cause him some pain.*

So far in the lesson the teacher's primary role has been to establish the lesson climate. That is, she informed the students about how they would be working and used silence to indicate to the students that it was their responsibility to initiate and carry the discussion. She took action to maintain the lesson structure when the structure broke down — when several students began talking at the same time. She sought to understand students by clarifying when she did not, and acknowledging when she did. When the students requested data, Ms. Pollock made it available when she was able to do so.

Since the discussion seemed well under way, Ms. Pollock felt the time was right to begin helping the students move toward the goals for values awareness lessons. In doing so, she looked for those moments during the student's discussion which would be appropriate for her to use some teaching behaviors specifically intended to yield the lesson goals. The discussion continues.

MS. POLLOCK: *Okay Daphne. You just reported a prediction about what might happen if he doesn't get some kind of treatment.*

DAPHNE: *Yeah.*

CARLTON: *I think the first thing Gerry should do is check in with a clinic or see a doctor as soon as possible to take care of the gonorrhea.*

FLOSSY: *You mean he shouldn't tell his girlfriend?*

CARLTON: *All I was saying was that he should get going on the treatment right away. He's right there in the doctor's office.*

MS. POLLOCK: *Uh-huh. That's something he could do.*

JACK: *I think one thing for sure is he ought to tell any girl he's had contact with.*

MS. POLLOCK: *Jack, would you be willing to share why you feel that way?*

JACK: *Well, I think he has the responsibility to any girls he's had contact with to tell them. He might have given it to them or caught it from one of them and they might not know they have it. Anyway, he should let them know. That's what he should do and maybe he can help keep some other people from getting it.*

MS. POLLOCK: *Jack, let me try something and you help me understand if this is what you're saying. It seems to me that one of your values about people is that they behave responsibly toward others, especially where diseases are involved. Did I catch it?*

JACK: *I never thought about it that way. Yeah... I do think people should let others know about those kinds of things instead of being ashamed or something and not telling them. That's not right.*

MS. POLLOCK: *Okay Jack.*

FERN: *A while ago somebody said that the doctor or clinic doesn't have to tell your parents if you have venereal disease. So, I think he should get the treatment, tell his girlfriend — girlfriends — but not tell his parents.*

MS. POLLOCK: *What do you think might happen, Fern, if he does what you said?*

FERN: *He'd get better and his girlfriend would too if she gets treated and his father wouldn't be disappointed with him.*

MS. POLLOCK: *His mother and father wouldn't be disappointed?*

FERN: *Right, like most parents if they thought you had a venereal disease.*

MS. POLLOCK: *Okay Fern.*

LEE: *I agree with Fern that he should take the treatment but not tell his parents because if he told his parents then they might not trust him or let him go out afterwards, or anything like that, because they might be afraid that he'd do the same thing over again. So, if he didn't tell his parents then he wouldn't be like grounded all the time for the rest of his life.*

MS. POLLOCK: *Then you're agreeing with Jim?*

LEE: *Yeah.*

MS. POLLOCK: *You're making a value judgment that that's a better approach as Fern said. Lee, can you think of any circumstances or conditions in which it would be a good idea to tell his parents?*

LEE: *Yeah, if he were to have a lot of guilt by not telling his parents then I think he should tell them.*

MS. POLLOCK: *All right.*

In these few illustrative student-teacher interactions drawn from an actual classroom lesson, it is apparent that Ms. Pollock's lesson was more than an open-ended discussion or rap session. In a good open-ended discussion the teacher may not participate at all other than setting up the discussion and posing the question for the discussion. In a values awareness lesson, however, the teacher must be able to systematically make those interventions intended to facilitate values awareness without interrupting or otherwise interfering with the integrity of the discussion. Thus, the teacher must not only know what interventions to make and when they should be made, but it is also critical that the teacher know how to make those interventions so the discussion will not become teacher dominated or teacher directed.

As in the case of most values awareness lessons, the implementation phase of the lesson concluded with a short Process Dialogue. At this time, Ms. Pollock invited the students to respond to questions such as:

How do you feel about the discussion we just had?

How can you deal with a person who seems to be monopolizing the discussion?

While there is a wide range of questions that may have been posed in a process dialogue, Ms. Pollock used these because she felt they were most relevant to what had happened among members of the class during the discussion. Naturally, she posed the first question and allowed the students adequate time to think and express themselves before going on to the second question.

A Glimpse — Some Disclaimers

The glimpse of a values awareness lesson provided on the preceding pages was presented so the reader would be able to get some feeling for both the climate of the lesson as well as what the teacher did to deliberately take some action toward the goals of values awareness. Certainly the actual discussion was more lengthy than the script provided. More students were involved and the teacher utilized several teaching behaviors in addition to those presented.

While Ms. Pollock used a transparency as a way to set the stage for the discussion question that would help students become aware of their values about social responsibility in relation to communicable diseases, a similar discussion might have been initiated in other ways. For example, a film, filmstrip, short story, newspaper article, or class or group activity that may deal with communicable diseases could have been used to set the stage for the discussion topic. For this lesson, Ms. Pollock involved the entire class in the discussion. Similar discussions could have been held with smaller groups of students as well. And, though this question was appropriate for Ms. Pollock's junior high students, a question such as, "How do you feel about people who don't cover their mouth when they sneeze?" would probably be more appropriate for primary grade students.

There is little doubt that having the proper classroom equipment and materials is important, as is adequate classroom facilities that make classroom discussions feasible. However, a values awareness lesson is more than equipment, materials, and facilities. The most crucial aspect of the lesson is the teacher. And the teacher is what the teacher does and does not do as he or she interacts with students.

Goals of the Values Awareness Teaching Strategy

One way to get a flavor of what a values awareness lesson is like is to observe a lesson or review a lesson script. Another way is to consider the goals intrinsic to these kinds of lessons. Following is a list of the goals of the Values Awareness Teaching Strategy.

The Values Awareness Teaching Strategy is intended to develop students':

- Awareness that the decisions they make are based in part on the values they hold.
- Awareness of the role of data in decision making.
- Awareness of the processes they or others use during a discussion and the effects of those processes on others.
- Awareness of some of the values they hold.
- Ability to systematically explicate their own values.
- Ability to systematically infer the values of others.
- Ability to analyze the source of data as one way of judging the validity of that data.
- Ability to weigh possible/probable consequences before implementing a course of action.
- Ability to recognize when they or others in a discussion are shifting topics.

- Ability to use language patterns that enable them to disagree with others while maintaining open lines of communication.
- Ability to interact effectively with others whose values differ.
- Ability to communicate their feelings, opinions and attitudes effectively.
- Ability to explicate the conditions that affect (1) the successful implementation of a course of action or (2) the prioritization of one's values.
- Awareness of the role of conditions in decision making.

Students' growth toward these goals takes place in three ways. First, for some students, participation in the discussion alone provides experiences that lead to the achievement of several of these goals. A second and perhaps more predictable way of facilitating students' growth is what the teacher does during the discussion. Finally, another significant element in facilitating students' growth toward some of these goals is the Process Dialogue following the discussion. It is obvious, though, that these goals are not achieved as a result of one or two values awareness lessons at the beginning of a semester. For most students, these goals are accomplished as an outgrowth of many values awareness lessons throughout their elementary and secondary school lives.

9

Teaching Behaviors Related to the Values Awareness Teaching Strategy

Teaching toward values awareness is effective to the degree that the teacher knows what she or he is doing and does it on purpose.

The most crucial element of any classroom is the teacher. It is what the teacher does and does not do that determines what the students will learn. Of course, having the kinds of facilities which make it possible for the teacher to group students in a variety of ways is important. In addition, the students and teachers must have audiovisual equipment and the necessary materials and supplies to work with. And most certainly, both teachers and students need a pleasant place to work so they can give their full attention to the matters at hand. It is difficult, if not impossible, to find any evidence which suggests that learning is more efficient, more effective, or that students feel better about themselves under such conditions alone. It is the teacher that counts; and the teacher is what the teacher does and does not do.

The Values Awareness Teaching Strategy is based on the premise that teaching is more effective if the teacher knows what she or he is doing and does it on purpose. Apart from the few in the teaching profession who are "born teachers," knowing what we are doing can make us more powerful. In a way, it is like touch typing versus the hunt and peck approach. Some people use the hunt-'n-peck approach and get by okay. In general, however, it is those people who have developed their skills related to the touch typing approach who can make that typewriter really "smoke."

Teaching is more than a mystical "either you've-got-it-or-you-haven't" art. Good teaching rests on some identifiable concepts and skills that can be studied, practiced, and mastered. In other words, people can learn what to do as teachers to facilitate their students' learning and they can learn when to do those things. Such are the prerequisites in teaching toward values awareness. What a teacher does as she or he interacts with students is referred to as a teaching behavior. A teaching behavior is a word, set of words, or some nonverbal actions used by the teacher which is intended to have some specified effect on the student's behavior or on student-student or student-teacher relationships.

In general, teaching behaviors related to most goals for instruction may be grouped into three categories. There are the *Basic Teaching Behaviors* through which the teacher creates and maintains the structure and integrity of the lesson. There are the *Goal Directed Teaching Behaviors* through which the teacher facilitates the student's growth toward the lesson objectives. And, there are the *Diagnostic Teaching Behaviors* the teacher uses as one way to generate data about the growth of the students toward those goals.

Deciding which teaching behavior to be used at any moment during a lesson is based on what the students do and where they are in their development toward the lesson goals. What words or actions are used to implement a specific teaching behavior is a professional decision guided by the teacher as an individual, the specific students with whom the teacher is working, classroom conditions, the relationship of today's lesson to what has preceded it and what will follow, and so on.

It is also important to point out that the Values Awareness Teaching Behaviors outlined in this material may be utilized in any setting whenever values awareness is a goal. Whether it is a total class lesson, a small group activity, a simulation, a game, a role playing situation, or an informal student-teacher dialogue in the classroom or on the playground, it is the teaching behavior utilized that determines whether or not students will become aware of the values they hold. Mere involvement in some classroom activity or discussion alone just does not do it. It is what the teacher does that determines what the students will learn.

The Basic Teaching Behaviors

The success of any lesson is dependent in part on how effectively the teacher is able to establish and maintain the integrity and structure of the lesson and the students' psychological freedom. By *integrity* and *structure* we mean that all of the students are dealing with the same issue in a thoughtful and responsible way. By *psychological freedom* we mean individual students in the group participate to the degree they want to as they (1) comment when they choose to do so or refrain from making comments when they choose; (2) respond to questions directed to them or "pass" for the time being; (3) agree or disagree with what others in the group have said; or (4) decide what data, if any, they need, and reach out to generate that data. The means whereby these classroom conditions are established and maintained are the *Basic Teaching Behaviors.* These teaching behaviors are:

- Structuring.
- Focus Setting.
- Clarifying.
- Acknowledging.
- Responding To Student's Data.
- Generating.
- Teacher Silence.

Each of these teaching behaviors is now described in detail.

Structuring

A critical element of all lessons is informing or reminding the students about how they will be working. One purpose of the Structuring teaching behavior is to do just that as the teacher initiates the lesson. Through this teaching behavior the teacher also lets the students know what the teacher expects of them and what they can expect of their teacher.

TEACHER: *Here's what we're going to do. I'm going to present a topic for you to discuss. As we work, it will be up to you to join in on the discussion on your own; I'm not going to call on anyone. If you have something you want to say, you can either just speak out when you get the opportunity or raise your hand and I'll call on you. Remember, though, let's have only one person talk at a time.* (And so on to complete the structuring as necessary for the lesson.)

In essence, the Structuring teaching behavior is the means the teacher uses to establish a climate that supports student-teacher and student-student communications by getting expectations and role relationships out in the open. Following is a list of the elements of the structure for a Values Awareness lesson that should be communicated to students who are to participate in this kind of a lesson for the first time.

TEACHER: *In our discussion today, I'm not going to call on you. You're going to let me know when you want to say something and you don't have to say anything unless you want to.*

If you have an opinion or idea about the topic, we'd like you to share it with us if you want to do so.

Sometimes you may not understand what someone is saying and you want to. It's okay to ask the person to repeat what he said or to ask him to say more about it.

It's okay to disagree with someone in the group, but it's out-of-bounds to attack them personally or to put them down.

Incidentally, if anyone in the group asks you a question, whether it's me or another student, you don't have to respond unless you are willing to do so.

Because this is a group discussion, it's important that all members of the group are able to hear what is said, so we'll ask that only one person speak at a time.

At times you may want to respond to something someone else in the group said. That's okay. You can talk to other people in the group, but remember, only one person talks at a time.

Any questions? I want you to feel comfortable in discussing the topic as you see it.

Here is a topic to which you might want to respond .... Focus Setting teaching behavior.

Of course, as students gain experience in working in this kind of lesson structure, structuring for a Values Awareness lesson could conceivably become:

TEACHER: *Today, we're going to work as we did last Thursday when.....*

So far we have reviewed the use of a Structuring teaching behavior to establish the lesson climate at the beginning of the lesson. The Structuring teaching behavior is also used during the lesson to maintain the established lesson structure. One element of the structure for a Values Awareness lesson is that the students initiate their own comments willingly. If the teacher judges that a student feels pressured to respond to a particular question from the teacher or from another student, for example, a Structuring teaching behavior is used to relieve the pressure on the student.

FRANK: *I don't know, maybe we should just go ahead and do what Francis said.*

TEACHER: *I'm not sure what you mean, Frank, are you saying we should all get together in our thinking and then go see the principal about it?* (Francis's course of action.)

FRANK: Looks confused or bewildered.

TEACHER: (Using structuring) *You can think about that and let me know if you want to say more, Frank. Okay?*

During the course of the lesson, Betty turns to Mildred and says:

BETTY: *Mildred, why do you think that companies that pollute the environment should be punished?*

MILDRED: Mildred's face flushes, she looks uneasy and does not respond.

TEACHER: *Mildred, you can pass on Betty's question if you'd like. If you want to respond later, that's okay. You can respond when you're ready.*

The Structuring teaching behavior is also used to maintain the lesson structure in those instances in which one student "puts down" another student.

BOB: *You know, I think you can get as much nutrition from one of those new instant breakfasts as you can from cereal, eggs, bacon, milk, toast, and juice.*

JAMIE: *Oh, come on. You sound like a salesman from one of those companies that lives off of peoples' stupidity. You're either an idiot, dumb, or both.*

TEACHER: *I want to remind you that those kinds of comments are not helpful in this kind of discussion. It's okay to disagree with Bob's idea, but putting him down either closes off a free sharing of ideas or can start an argument. At any rate, it doesn't help us get on the discussion.*

The Structuring teaching behavior is also used to restate or reinforce the lesson structure for the entire group when that structure breaks down.

CLASS: Several members of the group begin talking to each other while Francesca is speaking.

TEACHER: *Excuse me a minute, Francesca. Hold on there folks. We can't hear what's going on. Let's keep the discussion down to one person at a time otherwise we can't hear what anyone is saying.*

It is important to note that when a Structuring teaching behavior is used to deal with any breakdown in the lesson structure, it's recommended that a rationale for that structure also be reported to the students as in the foregoing examples, *"...putting him down either...," "....otherwise we can't hear...."*

A third purpose for the Structuring teaching behavior is to add to or modify the lesson structure established at the beginning of the lesson:

CLASS: Several members of the group begin talking to each other while Francesca is speaking.

TEACHER: *Excuse me, Francesca, would you hold what you want to say for a couple of minutes?* (Speaking to the entire group.) *It seems as though you people want to talk to each other about the topic in small groups. Why don't we take a few minutes to do that, then we'll get back to our group discussion and let Francesca continue.*

In summary, there are three different ways to use the Structuring teaching behavior. First, it is the way the teacher initiates the lesson by communicating how students will work, what the teacher expects of them, and what they can expect of their teacher. The Structuring teacher behavior also is used to maintain the lesson structure when that structure deteriorates. Finally, a Structuring teaching behavior is used to modify the lesson structure established by the teacher at the beginning of the lesson.

Focus Setting

One critical element of all lessons is informing students about what they will be working on. The purpose of the Focus Setting teaching behavior is to establish an explicit common topic or issue for discussion. Since there are different circumstances when this teaching behavior is used, there are different ways it may be formulated.

One way a Values Awareness lesson is initiated is as the teacher does Focus Setting by presenting a topic, usually in the form of a question, to the group for their discussion.

TEACHER: *One topic you may want to discuss is, "How do you feel about admission policies of college and universities which have been changed in order to encourage the enrollment of minorities and women?"*

TEACHER: *Following their mother's death, should Bill and Nancy's grandmother move in with them and their father?*

TEACHER: *How do you feel about people who sell dangerous drugs to their friends?*

The teacher might also use such a Focus Setting teaching behavior to restate the original question during the lesson or to shift to a new discussion topic either because the students have exhausted the original question or because the students did not have very much to say about it.

On occasion, as students participate in a discussion stimulated by the original Focus-Setting question, some may inadvertently begin to shift to a different unstated topic. This becomes apparent when their comments seem unrelated to the original Focus-Setting question. When this happens, a Focus Setting teaching behavior is used. In this case, the teaching behavior is intended to help the student become aware of the shift in topic she or he has made.

Original Focus-Setting Question:

Remember, Gerald has gonorrhea. Here's a question I'd like to invite you to respond to: "What do you think Gerald should do?"

After several students have responded to this topic by reporting what they think Gerald should do, Janet entered the discussion.

JANET: *I think the County Health Department should put people who get VD into a hospital and release them only when they are cured. That should help stop the spread.*

TEACHER: *Okay, Janet. You know, it seems as though you've shifted the original topic a bit. It sounds as though you are talking about the question, "What should other people do about people who get VD?"*

While in the foregoing example, the student shifted the discussion topic unknowingly, there are instances when a student may do so knowingly. The Focus Setting teaching behavior is used in this case to affirm that the student did indeed suggest a new or different topic for discussion.

SHIRLEY: *I know we've been talking about VD, but they can cure that. I really think a more important problem we ought to discuss is, "What should be done about the increasing teenage pregnancies?"*

TEACHER: *Yes, Shirley, that is another topic.*

Consequently, as in the case of the Structuring teaching behavior, there are three different ways the Focus Setting teaching behavior is used. In one instance the teacher presents a topic to be discussed. In the second case, the teacher interprets an unstated topic or question to which a student is responding that is different from the current topic of the discussion and states it for the student. In the third case, the teacher labels a discussion question presented by a member of the group as a new or different topic or issue.

Clarifying

A cornerstone of an effective Values Awareness lesson is effective student-teacher, teacher-student, and student-student communication. Good communication, however, is more than the expression of ideas, opinions, etc.; it also includes someone trying to understand what is being said. From the student's vantage point, therefore, a major purpose of a Values Awareness lesson is to give them an opportunity to express their ideas, feelings, opinions, values or attitudes about a given issue.

As students participate in a Values Awareness lesson, the teacher tries to understand the substance of the message they are communicating because he or she is interested. It is also important to understand what students are saying in order to determine how well the students are relating to the topic of the discussion. One purpose in using a Clarifying teacher behavior is therefore, to invite a student to help the teacher better understand the substance or content of the student's comment. Where possible, the Clarifying teaching behavior should give the student some indication of what it is that the teacher does not understand. In addition, it should be formulated in a way that puts the burden on the teacher for not being able to understand rather than to imply the student is dumb or stupid because he can not express himself effectively.

TEACHER: *Franella, help me understand what you mean by, "Mankind is an endangered species."*

TEACHER: *Could you say more about that, Tom?*

TEACHER: *I'm sorry, Wilma. I couldn't hear you. Would you please repeat that?*

TEACHER: *You've talked about several things, Ben. Are you saying that he should get treatment first and then decide whether or not to tell his parents?*

In order to be able to prescribe and use the range of teaching behaviors useful in facilitating Values Awareness, the teacher must be able to recognize or identify the specific student behavior occurring each time a student speaks. Another purpose a teacher might have for using a Clarifying teaching behavior even though she or he understands the substance of the student's message, therefore, is to enable the teacher to recognize the specific student behavior utilized. Consider the following student's comment:

DENNIS: *If we do what Mona suggests and stop all production of oil, our country would fall apart.*

At first glance it seems that Dennis is making a prediction. However, his intent might really be to disagree with Mona's suggestion and report a value judgment. Thus, the teacher uses a Clarifying teaching behavior to find out for sure.

TEACHER: *Dennis, help me understand. Are you making a prediction about what you feel might occur if Mona's suggestion was followed, or are you mainly disagreeing with her suggestion?*

In review, there are two purposes for using a Clarifying teaching behavior. First, the most frequent use is to enable the teacher to more fully understand what the student is saying — the substance of his or her message. A second purpose is to make it possible for the teacher to identify the specific student behavior. That is, is the student reporting a prediction, reporting data, making a value judgment, proposing a course of action, or what? When used for either of these purposes, the Clarifying teaching behavior should always be formulated in a "please help me to understand" context.

We note that the two expressed purposes for using this teaching behavior do not include helping one student understand what another student has said. While these kinds of teaching behaviors are necessary to some other teaching strategies, they are inconsistent with the goals and structure for a values awareness lesson in that they violate the students' psychological freedom.

Acknowledging

One aspect of effective communication is to let the person speaking know when you do not understand. Another aspect of equal importance is to let the person know when you do understand what they have said. The purpose in using an Acknowledging teaching behavior is to let a student who is talking to the teacher know that the teacher understands what she or he is saying.

Unlike some of the other teaching behaviors, this teaching behavior can be implemented through nonverbal as well as verbal means.

TEACHER: *I see.*

TEACHER: *Okay.*

TEACHER: *Uh-huh.*

TEACHER: Nods in acknowledgment.

TEACHER: *All right.*

While the Acknowledging teacher behavior is primarily used to let a student know the teacher understands the content of his or her message, it may also be used to acknowledge students' expression of feelings.

RALPH: *Boy, seeing drugs advertised on TV really gets me mad. It's as though they're trying to get kids and people popping drugs anytime things don't go the way they want.*

TEACHER: *I can see that you'd feel that way, Ralph.*

In summary, like Clarifying, the Acknowledging teaching behavior plays a fundamental role in student-teacher and teacher-student communication. It is the means whereby the teacher lets a student know his or her message is clear; that he or she is worthwhile and had made a contribution. If this intended effect is to be achieved, the way an Acknowledging teaching behavior is worded and when it is and is not used must be carefully considered. To use Acknowledging only when the teacher understands and agrees, but to do something else when the teacher understands and disagrees is to have seriously misunderstood the purpose and function of this teaching behavior. It is intended to be a nonjudgmental way of saying, "I understand."

In some instances when a teacher begins using the Values Awareness teaching strategy, she or he may be concerned that the students misread the Acknowledging teaching behavior and interpret it as "I agree." If this is a concern, it may be advisable for the teacher to use a Structuring teaching behavior to inform the students that when he or she makes a statement like, "I understand," "Okay," "Uh-huh," or nods, it only means he or she understands. It does not mean the teacher agrees with or disagrees with what the student has said.

Responding to Student's Data Generating

On occasion, during a discussion, people feel the need to generate some data. The same is true of students engaged in a Values Awareness lesson. For many, having access to the data is crucial to their continuing participation and intensity of involvement. The purpose of the Responding to Student's Data Generating teaching behavior is for the teacher to take some action to enable a student to get the data he or she needs. This may happen as the teacher gives a student the data requested, as the teacher identifies a data source the student can use, or by making it possible for the student to gain access to a data source identified.

TEACHER: *Ray, according to the information contained in one study, I know that about 45 percent of the students reported they started to smoke because all their friends smoked.*

TEACHER: *John, I really don't know how Blacks feel about the Sickle Cell anemia issue. Perhaps some of the students in this class who are in the Black Studies Program may want to respond to that question.*

MARGO: *I need to know what the state law requires as far as VD treatment.*

TEACHER: *Okay Margo, I'll make arrangements with Mrs. Lindburg, our nurse, so you can go in and use her copy of the State Health and Safety Code to find out about the VD laws.*

Though used less frequently than the Clarifying and Acknowledging teaching behaviors, the Responding to Student's Data Generating teaching behavior allows students to reach beyond opinions, feelings, and attitudes to bring some data to bear on the discussion. This teaching behavior is only used in response to individual students who have identified the data they need or the data source they want to utilize. It is not the intent of this teaching behavior to allow the teacher to provide data for a student that the teacher feels the student needs (though the student does not know it) to "straighten out his or her thinking" or to support a student's position with which the teacher agrees.

Teacher Silence

One of the conditions necessary for an effective values awareness lesson is that the students recognize it is their responsibility to initiate and carry the discussion. The purpose of the Teacher Silence teaching behavior is to communicate this idea to the students through nonverbal means.

In actual practice, this teaching behavior is not teacher silence alone, but is used by the teacher as a way of responding when there is student silence — when members of the group just sit there. In one sense, this teaching behavior is a nonbehavior!

STUDENTS: *(Silence)*

TEACHER: *(Silence)*

The Values Awareness Goal Directed Teaching Behaviors

The primary effect of the Basic Teaching Behaviors is to establish and maintain a classroom climate for values awareness. A classroom climate alone, however, does not facilitate the achievement of the goals for values awareness, except by chance. A few students get where we're going no matter what teachers do. The primary effect of the Values Awareness Goal Directed teaching behaviors is to facilitate the student's growth toward goals for Values Awareness lessons for the masses of students who would not achieve those goals by themselves. In one sense, all of the Values Awareness Goal Directed Teaching Behaviors are interventions. With a relevant and appropriate topic identified and the Basic Teaching Behaviors utilized correctly, the students will usually participate in a discussion. At selected appropriate moments during that discussion, the teacher uses various Values Awareness Goal Directed teaching behaviors with individual students in the group. The difficult task, however, is to know which of the Values Awareness Goal Directed teaching behaviors to use, to know when to use them, and to be able to use them to facilitate the students' growth toward the lesson goals in a way that does not interfere with the integrity and flow of the discussion for the students.

The Values Awareness Goal Directed teaching behaviors are:

- Tuning In To Process.
- Probe For Rationale.
- Inferring Value.

- Probe For Prediction.
- Probe For Data.
- Probe For Data Source.

Each of these teaching behaviors is now described in detail.

Tuning In To Process

People who participate in discussions can be more effective to the degree that they know what they are doing, can anticipate the probable effect of their own behavior on others, and do what they are doing on purpose. One purpose of the Tuning In To Process teaching behavior is to help the students become aware of what they are doing as they participate in value loaded discussions.

This teaching behavior may be used with an individual student or directed toward the entire group. When used with an individual student, the teacher simply and almost incidentally labels the behavior the student used.

> JOHN: *I think we'd solve the problem if there would be no more "cuts" into the tetherball line.*
>
> TEACHER: *John, you've just suggested one course of action that our class might take.* (Used to help the student become aware that he reported a course of action.)

> FRANCINE: *I don't agree with what Ruben said.*
>
> TEACHER: *Francine, you just made a value judgment about what Ruben suggested.* (Used to help the student become aware that she reported a value judgment.)

> PATTY: *If everyone who doesn't smoke complained when people smoke around them, it wouldn't be long before the smokers wouldn't smoke in public places.*
>
> TEACHER: *You just made a prediction about what you think would happen, Peggy.* (Used to help the student become aware that she reported a prediction.)

> MARY: *One of those articles sent out by the National Dairy Council states that milk is one of the most complete foods.*
>
> TEACHER: *That's some data you reported, Mary, about the food value of milk.* (Used to help the student become aware that she had reported some data.)

> FERGUSON: *Everybody here please raise your hand if you agree with this statement, "I would feel comfortable working for a boss who is a woman."*
>
> STUDENTS: Some class members hold up their hands.
>
> TEACHER: *Fergi, you just polled the class as a way of generating some data about their feelings about having a woman as a boss.* (Used to help the student become aware that he had generated some data.)

When directed toward an individual student, the Tuning In To Process teaching behavior helps the student become aware of his or her behavior at the moment. When directed toward a group, a second purpose of the Tuning In To Process teaching behavior is achieved: sensitizing the students to what is happening among members of the group.

TEACHER: *You know, as I listen to what most of the people in the group are saying, it seems that the emphasis of your comments is to make value judgments about the topic.*

TEACHER: *It's interesting to look at what has happened as we've been discussing this topic. First, everyone was against it, but now most of the people changed their minds, is that right?*

In review, the Tuning In To Process teaching behavior is the means the teacher uses both to help the students become aware of their behavior as individuals and to sensitize them to what is happening with the group. The Tuning In To Process teaching behavior should be used with caution when directed to the group because it may cause the group to shift from a discussion of the topic to a discussion of how they are working. This kind of shift is okay, as long as the teacher is aware of it.

Once students know what they are doing as they participate in a discussion and when they become attuned to the group as a whole, this teaching behavior will have achieved its purpose. There will be little need to use the Tuning In To Process teaching behavior with those students any longer. As a result, the terminology, "course of action," "value judgment," etc., becomes a part of the ongoing dialogue among students and the teacher.

Probe for Rationale

When involved in a discussion, people frequently make value judgments or propose courses of action. Less frequently, they report their rationale for those comments. Yet, it is an individual's rationale that offers the best clue to the values which underlie his or her value judgment or the course of action proposed. The purpose of the Probe for Rationale teaching behavior, therefore, is to invite a student to consider and report the bases he or she used in formulating a course of action or in making a value judgment.

TEACHER; *Penelope, what is your thinking behind your suggestion that we take money from our class treasury to buy a couch for the hallway outside the Principal's office?*

TEACHER: *Would you feel comfortable in sharing your reasons why you said it would be "good" to legalize abortions?*

TEACHER: *Tell me, Franklin, why do you say the sale of trail motorcycles ought to be against the law in our states?*

As with other probes, the Probe for Rationale teaching behavior should only be used in those instances in which the teacher is relatively certain the student will be able to respond and is willing to do so. In addition, the teaching behavior should be phrased in a way that does not demand or require a response from the student.

Inferring Value

One of the principal goals of the Values Awareness Teaching Strategy centers on helping students become aware of their values. Learning to become aware of one's values is best facilitated through social dialogue. For a teacher working with a group of students, the key tool of the teacher useful in fostering this awareness is the Inferring Value teaching behavior. The purpose of this behavior is to help the students become aware of the values that appear to be the bases for a course of action or value judgments they reported.

The Inferring Value teaching behavior is a set of words which (1) specify what the value is; (2) label the value as such; and (3) specify the subject of the value — that to which the value is applied. It is used only in those instances when the teacher understands a course of action reported or value judgment made by a student. In addition, the teacher must also know the student's rationale. Given these two kinds of information, the teacher will frequently be able to formulate an Inferring Value teaching behavior about the student's value(s). Whether the teacher does so or not will depend on what he or she knows about whether the student will feel free to restate what the teacher has said or even disagree with the values inferred.

In order to insure that the student will feel free to disagree with, add to or modify what the teacher has said, the Inferring Value teaching behavior is always formulated in an "It seems to me..." "Would you agree that..." "It looks as though..." context. Furthermore, it is phrased and communicated through words carefully chosen, voice inflection, and general body language that invites students to respond freely and on their own terms.

TEACHER: *It seems to me — and help me if I'm off course — that one of your values about families is that they provide a feeling of belonging for members. Did I understand you correctly?*

TEACHER: *Based on what you just said, Ripley, would it be fair to say that one of your values about families is that they are a source of support for those in the family?*

In view of the fact that the way this teaching behavior is used is critical to the success of the lesson, (to use it incorrectly might make students feel the teacher is attempting to put words in their mouth rather than help them gain insight into themselves) an entire chapter is devoted to the use of the Inferring Value teaching behavior. That chapter is entitled, "Individualizing the Use of the Inferring Teaching Behavior."

Probe for Prediction

One of the goals common to all health educators is getting students in the habit of considering the consequences of their actions or decisions before they are implemented. Stated in another way, to consider possible consequences is to forecast data — to make a prediction. The purpose of the Probe for Prediction teaching behavior, therefore, is to invite students to consider possible consequences of a given course of action they recommend.

TEACHER: *Wilma, how do you think kids in the other classes might react if we were given the best playground area for the rest of the semester?*

TEACHER: *What do you predict the response will be if we have people sign their names to the drug survey rather than having it anonymous?*

TEACHER: *Tom, what do you think might happen if one were to take that approach; that is, how might the people involved feel about it?*

The teacher uses the Probe for Prediction teaching behavior to get the students thinking about consequences when they do not do so for themselves. Obviously, for those students who begin to give this kind of consideration to their decision making on their own, the teacher will no longer need to use this teaching behavior. Hopefully, as a result of using the Probe for Prediction teaching behavior students will find that the solutions to problems they implement will be more effective for them and less frequently create new problems.

Probe for Data

It is not uncommon for people to make decisions based on

opinions, feelings, attitudes, beliefs, or values alone. For many day-to-day decisions this base is adequate. For many other decisions, however, this base is inadequate. Data are also needed if the decision is to be a viable one. The purpose of the Probe for Data teaching behavior is to sensitize students to the need for and the effect of data on the decisions they make. In addition, this teaching behavior may also lead to the development of the student's ability to differentiate between judgments and decisions that are based in part on data from those based wholly on opinions, feelings, attitudes, beliefs, or values. This is not to suggest that one decision is better than the other, but only to help students become aware that the ways these decisions were formulated are different in that respect. Through the Probe for Data teaching behavior, the teacher invites the student to report data he or she has or needs to support a course of action, prediction, or value judgment.

TEACHER: *Charlene, what data would you need to decide if the course of action you just reported looks like it will work?*

TEACHER: *Betty, is your prediction based on any data you know about, or is it just what seems might happen?*

TEACHER: *Romero, do you know of any data you'd be willing to share that supports your judgment about the free clinic in our neighborhood?*

When used in response to a student who has reported a course of action, prediction, or value judgment, the Probe for Data helps sensitize students to the role of data in decision making. Certainly, like any of the other teaching behaviors, it should not be used each time these student behaviors occur. Furthermore, the teacher is cautioned not to fall into the habit of using this teaching behavior either, only in response to those student statements with which he or she agrees, or only in response to those student behaviors with which he or she disagrees. If used in these selected situations, the Probe for Data teaching behavior tends to cue students about the teacher's position about the issue under discussion rather than to achieve its intended effect.

Probe for Data Source

Working with data usually raises a question about data sources: "Where will I get the data I need?" The purpose of the Probe for Data Source teaching behavior is to help students expand their repertoire of data sources. When used before a student has taken any action to generate data, this teaching behavior both sensitizes him or her to the need for data as well as raising the issue of where he or she will get it.

TEACHER: *Vasquez, do you have any ideas about where you might get that information you want?*

When used some time after a student has generated data, the Probe for Data Source teaching behavior helps him or her become consciously aware of the data source used.

TEACHER: *I'm curious, Clancy, would you be willing to share where you got that data?*

TEACHER: *Did you get the data just reported from the Resource Center, from your friends, or from somewhere else?*

While the prime purpose in using a Probe for Data Source is to expand the student's repertoire of data sources he or she knows of, knowing where some data came from also enables an individual to make some estimates about the validity of the data as well. This experience can set the stage for Concept Development lessons about valid data and/or Skill Development lessons in which students learn to use various techniques of data validation.

The Values Awareness Diagnostic Teaching Behaviors

With many occupations, evidence of a job well done is readily apparent. An automobile mechanic takes pride in the sound of a well-tuned engine. A builder can step back and admire the structure created. A salesperson can boast of a quota met and satisfied customers. A physician feels competent as the patient recovers. But how does the teacher know the job is well done?

With some lessons, the answer to the teacher's concerns about a job well done is found in the student's ability to recall relevant information at the right time, demonstrate proficiency in a particular skill, or use a given concept to build an explanation or make a prediction. In values awareness lessons, the teacher watches for the occurrence of certain student behaviors. For example, students give evidence that they are aware of what is going on during a discussion as they incidentally label the various behaviors used in the discussion. Or, they may make a value statement in relation to their own values or the values of others. Or, they voluntarily specify the conditions under which they would support a given course of action or value judgment.

On occasion, students who are nearing the goals of values aware-ness may demonstrate these kinds of behaviors voluntarily during a lesson. More frequently, however, when students are deeply involved in a given topic or issue, their behavior may be limited to specific responses to the topic. Even though they are able to do so, evidence of growth toward the lesson goals sought by the teacher may not be demonstrated by the students. In such instances, the teacher can draw on the Values Awareness Diagnostic teaching behaviors.

The Values Awareness Diagnostic teaching behaviors are:

* Probe For Values.
* Probe For Process Awareness.
* Probe For Conditions.
* Probe For Feelings.

Each of these teaching behaviors is now described in detail.

Probe for Values

The central thrust of the Values Awareness Teaching Strategy is to help students gain insight into their own values, explicate their own values, or infer the values of others. When the teacher has used the Inferring Values teaching behavior with a student on several occasions over the course of several lessons, the teacher may want to take action to find out if the student is able to explicate her or his own values or infer the values of others if the student has not done so voluntarily.

During a discussion, the purpose of the Probe for Values teaching behavior is to invite the student to make a value statement about his or her own values or the values of someone else, depending on the context in which it is used. Furthermore, this teaching behavior is always directed to an individual student rather than to the class as a whole.

MANFRED: *I think everyone should take some time out during the day for physical exercise.*

TEACHER: *Manfred, would you be willing to share any of your values that lead you to make that statement?*

LUCY: *I agree with changing the law on abortion.*

TEACHER: *Okay Lucy. Would you feel comfortable in sharing some of your values that underlie the judgment you just made?*

TEACHER: *Based on what you just said about what Ronald McDonald liked about his friends, can you tell what some of his values about friends might be?*

It is important to note that the Probe for Values teaching behavior should only be used at that time when the teacher is relatively sure the student will be willing and able to formulate a values statement in response. Even in these instances when a student is unable to respond, (and the teacher uses a Structuring teaching behavior to make her or him feel free not to do so) the Probe for Values teaching behavior has a positive effect on the student. Because he or she wants to know what values are held, the student usually continues thinking about the question.

Probe for Process Awareness

In using the Tuning In To Process teaching behavior, the teacher takes action to help the students become aware of what they are doing as they participate in discussions about values related topics or issues. The purpose of the Probe for Process Awareness teaching behaviors is to enable the teacher to find out if students are becoming aware of what they are doing when they have not given evidence of such awareness on their own.

While most frequently, this teaching behavior is used with an individual student in relation to his or her own behavior, it may also be used with an individual student in relation to what is going on with other members of the group or it may be used with the group as a whole.

TEACHER: *Tell me, Clem, when you said, "The dress code is unfair," do you know what it was you did?*

WALLA: *I think that if you got rid of all the ash trays in public buildings like Johnny said, that would stop the smoking there.*

TEACHER: *Okay Walla.* (Pause) *What would you call that statement you just made?*

TEACHER: *Hey, would anyone like to comment about what just happened in the group?*

FARQUARDT: *Yeah, we just shifted to a different topic. We started out talking about our feelings about the use of marijuana and now we're talking about what the Mexican Government should do about the illegal poppy fields in the mountains.*

It is important to note that in those occasions when a student does not respond or when he or she does not respond appropriately to the

Probe for Process Awareness teaching behavior, the teacher should not take that opportunity to "correct" the student. Rather, it indicates the student is not yet fully aware of his or her behavior. The Tuning In To Process teaching behavior should be used in ensuing lessons while continuing to monitor the student's growth toward process awareness with the occasional use of the Probe for Process Awareness teaching behavior.

Probe for Conditions

At one level of values development, in recommending a course of action to be followed or in reporting a value judgment, students take a stand without regard for the specific circumstances that surround that situation. At a more sophisticated level of development, students seek out information about the conditions related to the problem or issue in order to account for them in the solution they propose. Unfortunately, however, they frequently fail to mention the specific circumstances or conditions they have considered as they participate in a values loaded discussion. The purpose of the Probe for Conditions teaching behavior is to invite the student to report the various conditions or factors he or she has considered which affect the successful implementation of a proposed solution.

TEACHER: *Franellippe, what are some of the conditions you considered in formulating your course of action about improving the nutritional value of the food in the cafeteria?*

TEACHER: *Would you be willing to share what conditions would affect your values about health insurance plans?*

TEACHER: *Under what circumstances would that course of action be the only one that would work?*

Depending on where a student is in his or her development, the Probe for Conditions teaching behavior may serve a purpose different from providing diagnostic information alone. For the student who has considered but not reported the various circumstances that surround the successful implementation of a problem solution she or he has proposed, this teaching behavior serves a diagnostic purpose by giving the teacher that information. For the student who has not given thought to such circumstances, this teaching behavior serves a diagnostic purpose by providing the teacher with that information. However, in this latter instance, the Probe for Conditions teaching behavior also frequently facilitates the student's growth toward values awareness goals by stimulating or alerting him or her to some conditions that may influence the successful resolution of the problem or issue.

Probe for Feelings

While all of the other teaching behaviors described are intended to either create and maintain a climate for the student's discussion, facilitate, or diagnose the students' growth toward the goals of values awareness, the Probe for Feelings teaching behavior serves a different purpose. The purpose of this teaching behavior is to give the teacher some direct affective feedback from the students about how they felt about the lesson. This teaching behavior is usually directed to the entire group rather than to an individual student.

The Probe for Feelings teaching behaviors may be used in relation to the lesson topic; *How do you feel about the topic we used for our discussion today?* about the way the group was organized; *How do you feel about how the class was organized for the lesson?* about how the lesson was structured; *How do you feel about how we worked today?* about how members of the group participated in the lesson, about the lesson in general, etc. While students' responses on such Probe for Feelings teaching behaviors are not necessarily diagnostic data about their growth, those responses do offer diagnostic data for the teacher about the student's affective response to the lesson.

TEACHER: *How do you feel about the subject we discussed today?*

TEACHER: *What do you think about our discussion today?*

TEACHER: *How do you feel about the way we've been working?*

TEACHER: *How do you feel about discussing the kinds of topics we've been considering during the last few days?*

TEACHER: *I notice that during this discussion, there are times when we have periods of silence — when no one is talking. How do you feel about that? Does it bother you in any way?*

Since this teaching behavior represents a departure from the specific discussion topic, it is usually used during the Process Dialogue portion of the discussion. It is always posed to the entire group so no individual student will feel as though she or he has been "put on the spot" to respond. The students' responses offer the teacher insight into their affective reactions to the lesson.

Teaching Behaviors Inconsistent with the Goals of Values Awareness

The discussion about teaching behaviors thus far has centered on what the teacher does to create a climate for values awareness lessons, to facilitate the student's growth toward values awareness goals, and to generate diagnostic data about the students' progress. What have not been discussed, however, are those teaching behaviors that interfere with the goals for values awareness lessons. In essence, any teaching behavior — anything a teacher does or says — which is intended to implement a teacher role not a part of the Values Awareness Teaching Strategy will probably be counter-productive to it. For example, some characteristic teacher roles in a Skill Development Teaching Strategy are to "provide feedback, positive reinforcement, and psychological support for the students as they work." To use any teaching behavior intended to implement either of these roles during a values awareness lesson would put the teacher in the position of favoring one opinion, attitude, or course of action over others. Since in doing so the teacher no longer maintains a neutral position in relation to the topic of the discussion, the climate necessary for an effective values awareness lesson may be endangered.

Other teacher roles inconsistent with the Values Awareness Teaching Strategy include, "guiding students by cueing and summarizing." The effect of cueing and summarizing is to get the students on the "right track" or let them know when they are "there." Obviously, to cue students or to summarize their responses during a values awareness lesson would be to tell the students directly or indirectly what the teacher feels their values should be. Since this is inconsistent with the climate, goals, and structure of values awareness lessons, these kinds of teaching behaviors are inappropriate.

It is clear that the basis used to determine if a given teaching behavior is appropriate or not is to consider the effect of that teaching behavior. If the effect of that teacher role is inconsistent with the teacher roles identified for the Values Awareness Teaching Strategy, the teaching behavior in question should probably not be used during the values awareness lesson.

10

Individualizing the Use
of the Inferring
Value Teaching Behavior

*In using the inferring value dialogue,
the teacher makes it possible for a student to communicate something of
whom he or she is — of what is important to him or her.*

Have you ever walked away from a conversation with someone
you have just met and thought, "What a neat person. They're really
interesting." On the other hand, you may have thought, "I'm sure glad
I don't have to work with them." Have you ever wondered how you
reached those judgments? The chances are that during your
conversation with them you intuited some of their values about the
subject of your discussion. In the first case, you had positive feelings
about the person probably because there was a match between the
values you intuited and your own values. In the other case, there was
probably a mismatch.

We intuit the values of others all the time. It's normal, it's
natural, and it's part of human interaction. However, one of the
shortcomings of this process is that all too frequently we may misread
the values of others and, consequently, misjudge them as people.

In our view, there are two reasons why this happens. First, we
assume our intuitive readings of the values of others are correct
without checking with the other person to see if they are indeed the
values he holds about the subject under discussion. A second reason
we misjudge people is that we seldom utilize a deliberate process that
yields adequate data as a base to infer their values. Which is a more
humane way to read the values of others, to rely solely on our
intuition, or add to that a process by which we can more accurately go
about building and testing this inference?

These notions about inferring values of others intuitively or through the use of a more deliberate process are more true of interactions in the classroom than they are outside of the classroom. The use of a deliberate process to infer values in the classroom is crucial when one of the teacher's objectives for values education is to help students become aware of their values. Such a process not only yields values awareness for students when used by the teacher, but more importantly, by involvement in the process it develops the student's ability to more accurately explicate his or her own values and to infer the values of others.

Using the Inferring Value Dialogue

The purpose of an Inferring Value Dialogue is for the teacher to formulate a value statement about the student's value(s) with which the student agrees. A value statement is defined as a set of words which:

- Specify what the value is.
- Label the value as such.
- Specify the subject of the value — that to which the value is applied.

For a set of words to be a value statement, all three components must be included though the sequence in which they occur is not important.

It is critical to note that there are two ways an individual can arrive at a value statement. One way occurs when an individual reflects on and reports his or her own value(s). For example, *One of my values about exercise is that it makes me feel good.* We refer to this as explicating one's value. The other way an individual may arrive at a value statement is to make an inference about a value of someone else. For example, *Based on what you've said La Lanne, it seems to me that one of the things you value about exercise is that it makes you feel good.* This is referred to as inferring someone's value when an individual reports one of his values, he knows the subject and his value(s) about the subject. However, when one person attempts to infer the value(s) of someone else, it is necessary to generate and check out the subject and the value through dialogue.

For the teacher who wants to use the Inferring Value teaching behavior, both components of a value statement, the value and the subject of the value, are generated for the teacher through the

Inferring Value Dialogue. An Inferring Values Dialogue is the systematic utilization of a sequence of teaching behaviors designed to move from the student's expression of a value judgment or a course of action to the identification of the value(s) that underlies that value judgment or course of action.

Because most value judgments and courses of action are based on values, it is possible to "read back" from them to the values which underlie these judgments or actions. Therefore, the starting point for the Inferring Values Dialogue is when a student reports a course of action or value judgment. However, since different people may make the same value judgment or propose the same course of action for different reasons, more information is necessary. A rationale is needed from the student which communicates why he or she has made a judgment or recommended a course of action. It is through both the value judgment or course of action along with the rationale offered by the student, that the subject of a value statement may be identified and the value inferred by the teacher.

Because inferences about the values of students are tentative at best, the teacher has the responsibility to use the Inferring Values teaching behavior in a manner that invites the student to respond to the teacher's statement. The student may respond by agreeing, disagreeing, making a modification, or by indicating a desire to think about it before responding.

What follows is a general outline of an Inferring Value Dialogue. This dialogue is discussed in a two-phase sequence. Phase I is called *Getting Ready*. It centers on identifying the subject and inferring the value. Phase II is called *Formulating and Using the Inferring Value Teaching Behavior*. It centers on the way the teacher formulates and uses the Inferring Value teaching behavior with students.

Phase I:
Getting Ready

Getting ready to formulate an Inferring Value teaching behavior involves inferring the value and identifying the subject of the value from either value judgments or courses of action and related rationale reported by students.

Focus-Setting Question: How do you feel about school this year?

PATRICIA: *I really like school this year because you get to pick some of the classes you take.*

—The value: *pick some classes.*
—The subject: *school this year.*

In this example both the value and subject of the value are clear so the teacher could move on to Phase II: *Formulating and Using the Inferring Value Teaching Behavior.*
In this example of Phase I of the Inferring Value Dialogue, Patricia voluntarily included a rationale for her position. The rationale followed the word "because." On occasion, however, students do not add their rationale to a value judgment or course of action voluntarily. To invite the student to share his or her rationale, a Probe for Rationale teaching behavior may be used.

Focus-Setting Question: How do you feel about school this year?

MAYNARD: *I really like it.*

TEACHER: *Would you be willing to share why you feel that way, Maynard?* (Probe for Rationale teaching behavior)

MAYNARD: *Because it's fun.* (Consider the Focus Setting to understand what the student means by "it.")

"Fun" is the student's rationale. However, since words like "fun," "nice," "good," and so on, are open to numerous interpretations, a Clarifying teaching behavior may be used to get the additional information necessary to infer the student's value.

TEACHER: *I'm not sure what you mean by "fun." Would you say some more about that?* (Clarifying teaching behavior).

MAYNARD: *Well, this year I get a chance to talk in class and to hear what other kids have to say.*

—The value: *Chance to talk and hear what others have to say. This may be translated to "chance to share ideas."*
—The subject of the value: *School this year.*

If after using the Clarifying teaching behavior, the value and/or subject of the value remains unclear, the teacher may just use the Acknowledging teaching behavior and not proceed with the Inferring Value Dialogue. Since students are responding to the topic of the Focus Setting as they make a value judgment or report a course of action, it may be easier to identify the subject of the student's value if the topic of the Focus Setting is kept in mind. Quite often in health related discussions, the subject of the student's value(s) is implicit in the student's comment. That is, the subject is frequently the student's own mental-emotional, social, or physiological state.

With the value inferred and the subject of the value identified, the teacher is ready to move to Phase II: *Formulating and Using the Inferring Value teaching behavior.*

Phase II: Formulating and Using the Inferring Value Teaching Behavior

The Inferring Value teaching behavior should be utilized only when the teacher feels relatively certain the value and subject of the value have been accurately inferred. An Inferring Value teaching behavior has three elements. These elements should:

• Specify what the value is.
• Label the value as such.
• Specify the subject of the value, that to which the value is applied.

The following is an example of the Inferring Value teaching behavior in which these elements are identified.

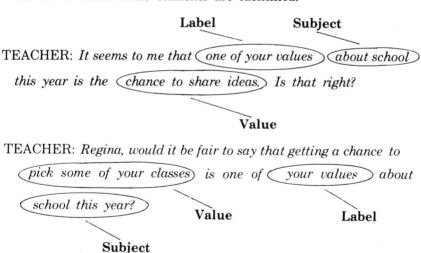

TEACHER: *It seems to me that one of your values about school this year is the chance to share ideas. Is that right?*

TEACHER: *Regina, would it be fair to say that getting a chance to pick some of your classes is one of your values about school this year?*

The Inferring Value teaching behavior must be expressed in a way that invites the student to question or disagree with what the teacher has said. This is necessary in order to clearly indicate to the student that you are trying to understand their values in order to help them become aware of those values rather than tell them what their values are or should be. It is for this reason that phrases such as those that follow are usually used as part of the Inferring Values teaching behavior.

- It sounds as though one of the things you're saying is... Is that what you're saying?
- Would it be fair to say that...?
- I kind of hear you saying... Is that what you're saying?
- I don't want to put words in your mouth so please correct me if I haven't understood you — it sounds like you're saying that... Is that right?
- Would it be accurate to say...?
- I'm getting the message that one of your values... Is that right?

If the student disagrees or does not understand, the teacher may reformulate the Inferring Value teaching behavior or use an Acknowledging teaching behavior and terminate the Inferring Value Dialogue. If the student appears to be confused, a Structuring teaching behavior should be used to let the student know he or she does not have to respond to the teacher at that time. The purpose in using this teaching behavior is to communicate that it is okay to think and to take all of the time necessary to do so.

An Example of the Inferring Value Dialogue

As a way to get a feeling for the flow and climate of an Inferring Value Dialogue, we will draw an example from a values awareness lesson in response to the educational telecast entitled "Travelin Shoes."** This telecast begins as Larry Billups has come to the hard decision that he must move his family from the country neighborhood where they have always lived to Washington, D.C. He knows that he needs to make a better living for them, although moving means giving up their relatives, old friends, their church, and the pleasures of the water. Stuart, his son, resists the whole idea, and tries to persuade his parents to let him stay with his grandfather. His older sister, Kim, can hardly wait to get to the city, where she expects to discover a more exciting kind of life. Didi, the youngest child, is a passive observer of the events that surround her. The Focus-Setting question posed by the teacher at the conclusion of the telecast was, *Should Stuart go with his family when they move to the city?*
    Various members of the group have responded to the question by presenting different courses of action they felt Stuart should follow.

** *This educational television program is part of the Inside/Out television series produced by Agency for Instructional Television, Bloomington, Indiana 1973.*

Other students reported data about the film or about some other families who had also experienced the need to move to a new location because of a change in their dad's job. Then Judie spoke. The teacher felt that this would be a good opportunity to implement the Inferring Values dialogue with Judie to help her become aware of some of her own values about a family.

JUDIE: *I think Stuart should go to the city with his family when they move.*

TEACHER: *Judie, would you feel comfortable in telling us why you think he should do that?*

JUDIE: *Yeah, because of all the help and care they'll give him as he's growing up.*

TEACHER: *I hear you saying that some of the values you hold about a family is that the family provides help and care for their kids, is that right?*

JUDIE: *Yeah, that's right.*

TEACHER: *Okay Judie.*

This is an example of an Inferring Value Dialogue. Now, let us revisit this dialogue step-by-step and consider what went on. First, Judie reports a course of action:

JUDIE: *I think Stuart should go to the city with his family when they move.*

Having heard a course of action but without a rationale, the teacher initiated the Inferring Value Dialogue with a Probe for Rationale teaching behavior. Obviously, if Judie had included a rationale in support of her course of action, this teaching behavior would not have been necessary.

TEACHER: *Judie, would you feel comfortable in telling us why you think he should do that?*

To which Judie responds with:

JUDIE: *Yeah, because of all the help and care they'll give him as he's growing up.*

The teacher saw the values expressed by Judie as "help" and "care." And it seemed that the subject of these values was "family" because that is to what the values "help" and "care" were applied.

With the values and the subject of the value identified, the teacher formulated and used the Inferring Value teaching behavior.

TEACHER: *I hear you saying that some of the values you hold about a family is that the family provides help and care for their kids. Is that right?*

You can see that the Inferring Value Dialogue centers on the Inferring Value teaching behavior. Any student-teacher interaction that precedes the use of this teaching behavior is intended to enable the teacher to identify the value and subject of the value in order to formulate the Inferring Value teaching behavior. In studying the Inferring Value teaching behavior you will note that the values were specified, "help" and "care," the values were labeled as such: "some of the values you hold...," and the subject of the values was specified as "family." Of course, the teacher could have elected to broaden the subject, "family," to "families," but she chose not to do so in this case. For an adult, values about the family may be that it meets the growing child's basic needs such as food, shelter, clothing, and love, that it provides a supportive environment, meets the child's spiritual needs, and so on. For Judie, the values surfaced about a family were "help" and "care." While these may not be the teacher's major values about a family or all of Judie's values about a family for that matter, they were the values surfaced in this dialogue. And Judie responded to the Inferring Value teaching behavior with:

JUDIE: *Yeah, that's right.*

And the teacher responds to Judie with an Acknowledging teaching behavior:

TEACHER: *Okay Judie.*

It is critical that the Inferring Value teaching behavior is expressed as a question in order to invite the student to respond. In those instances when a student responds with a comment like, "No, that's not exactly what I meant," that's an indication that the climate for the Values Awareness Teaching Strategy is working effectively. That is, the student feels comfortable in letting the teacher know that the teacher missed the student's point. As was mentioned earlier, when the teacher reads confusion or lack of agreement on the part of the student, the Inferring Value Dialogue may be terminated regardless of how well the teacher feels he or she understands the student's values. That student may not be ready or willing to talk about his or her values about that topic at that time. And, the student should not be put on the spot to do so. Drawing inferences about the values of others is a complex process and should be done very thoughtfully and carefully. Doing so should be attempted only in a classroom climate where the students recognize that the teacher is not trying to impose his or her values on them.

General Comments About the Inferring Value Dialogue

Broadening the Subject of the Value

In formulating the Inferring Values teaching behavior, the teacher may broaden the subject of the value expressed by the student to a more general category. For example, with a student's subject expressed as "school this year," the teacher may broaden it to "school." "Red Circle health plan" may be broadened to "health plans"; "dinner" may be broadened to "meals" or "food." In broadening the subject, the teacher is actually inviting the student to consider whether the value surfaced about the subject expressed is also a value the individual holds about the broader subject. Care should be exercised in broadening the subject so as not to broaden it too far beyond the subject the student is discussing. For example, broadening the subject "dinner" to "recommended daily food allowances" may lose the student.

Translating Values

In some instances when the student has used a lengthy or convoluted phrase to express a value, the teacher may find it useful to transform the phrase into more concise language. For example, "chance to talk in class and to hear what others say," may be changed to, "chance to share ideas." Care should be exercised in translating values to assure that the translation (1) is not too great a leap for the student to track, or (2) does not put words in the student's mouth.

Avoiding Teacher Dominated Dialogue

If at any point during the Inferring Value Dialogue the teacher feels the interaction is becoming teacher dominated, the dialogue should be terminated. An Acknowledging teaching behavior should be used to indicate "message received" and thereby relieve the pressure on the student to try to communicate something he or she may not be ready to at that time.

Stimulating Values Thinking

Even when the Inferring Value Dialogue is not successful in surfacing the student's values about a given subject, at least two positive outcomes usually result. First, the student feels the teacher is interested in him as a person because of the nature of the interaction itself. Second, it stimulates the student to continue thinking about the question, *"Just what are my values about...?"*

Dealing with Negative Rationales

On occasion, when students state a value judgment or course of action, the rationale used may outline nonpreferences or things they dislike. Since values are preferences, it is necessary for the teacher to infer preferences from the dislikes expressed. Or, the teacher may use a Clarifying teaching behavior to invite the students to indicate what their preferences actually are. The following is an example of the teacher inferring a preference from a nonpreference.

TEACHER: *How do you feel about people who smoke?*

JAMIE: *People who smoke are dumb.*

TEACHER: *Would you be willing to share why you feel that way?*

JAMIE: *If they keep it up, they'll probably get lung cancer.*

TEACHER: *Would it be fair to say that one of your values about not smoking is that it's one way of maintaining health?*

In this example the teacher inferred "maintaining health" as the value from the students' stated dislike, "get lung cancer." In this case as in other Inferring Value Dialogues, the teacher listens for agreement.

JAMIE: *Sure.*

A Summary of the Flow of an Inferring Value Dialogue

Phase I: Getting Ready

• When the student Reports a Value Judgment or Course of Action with a rationale
—listen for the value and the subject of the value.
• When the student Reports a Value Judgment or Course of Action without a rationale
—use a Probe for Rationale teaching behavior and listen for the value and subject of the value.

Phase II: Formulating and Using the Inferring Value Teaching Behavior

• Formulate and use the Inferring Value teaching behavior by
—specifying what the value is
—labeling the value as a value
—specifying the subject of the value. The subject of the value may
be translated as appropriate then,
• Listen for agreement.

11

Selecting and Presenting the Focus for a Values Awareness Lesson

Two events are necessary to initiate a values awareness lesson: informing students how they will be working and letting them know on what they will be working — what topic they will be discussing. Informing students how they will be working is referred to as a Structuring teaching behavior. To formulate a Structuring teaching behavior, the teacher has only to give some thought to what students are to do during the lesson, how they are to be organized, and what they can expect from their teacher.

Letting the students know what they will be discussing, using the Focus-Setting teaching behavior, on the other hand, takes much more planning and deliberation. In this case, the teacher must be able to identify a specific topic, phrase the discussion question, and in many instances, create the setting for the question that makes it "real" for the students. The purposes of this chapter are to provide criteria useful in formulating or selecting a Focus-Setting question and to suggest some general alternatives useful in setting the stage for these questions.

Three Criteria Useful in Selecting the Focus-Setting Question

A question that specifies the topic for a values awareness discussion is referred to as a Focus-Setting behavior. Either the teacher or the students can formulate a Focus-Setting behavior. While there are different questions a teacher or the students can pose in an attempt to stimulate a values awareness lesson, not just any question will do the job. The task for the teacher is to either formulate his or her own questions or select those questions from curriculum materials or those posed by the students that offer the greatest chances for a successful lesson. But how does the teacher recognize those questions? A careful analysis of focus-setting questions that produce lively and productive values awareness lessons has led to the identification of the following three criteria useful in formulating or selecting them.

Three Criteria

- Criterion No. 1: Is the topic of the focus-setting question within the knowledge of the students?

The extent of students' knowledge of a discussion topic is one factor that affects their participation in a values awareness lesson. Consider the discussion topic of fad diets, for example. Students who do not know what a fad diet is will probably have little to contribute to the discussion other than to ask questions about what a fad diet is. Their participation will probably be minimal at best. Students who have some knowledge of fad diets, because they may have heard about them on television, heard them discussed at home, or who have done some reading about them will, no doubt, have more to contribute. The chances are that they will participate more than their uninformed counterparts in the classroom. Of course the greatest participation may be anticipated from these students who have extensive knowledge about the subject. Such knowledge may have resulted from studying pros and cons about fad diets, talking to others who have used such diets, using a fad diet themselves, and so on.

The way one's knowledge about a topic affects their participation in a discussion about it is obvious. The more students know about the focus-setting question, the greater are the chances for the success of the lesson.

- Criterion No. 2: Is the focus-setting question relevant to the students?

Another factor that affects students' participation in a values awareness lesson is what we call the personal relevance of the particular discussion topic. In assessing personal relevance, the teacher makes a judgment about how meaningful the topic will be to the lives, interests, or concerns of his or her students. Consider the following topics, for example, in relation to a group of third grade students: (1) the behavior of adults at a recent city council hearing; (2) the behavior of teenagers at a recent rock concert; and (3) the behavior of third graders on the playground during recess. It seems obvious that the first topic will probably be irrelevant to most third graders. Because many third graders look forward to the time when they will attend a rock concert, the second topic may be somewhat relevant to them. It is clear that the third topic, their own behavior on the playground during recess, will probably be highly relevant for them.

The way the personal relevance of a particular discussion topic influences students' participation in a values awareness lesson is clear. The more the focus-setting question relates to the lives, interests, or concerns of students the more relevant it is. The more relevant it is, the greater the likelihood the lesson will be successful.

- Criterion No. 3: Is the focus-setting question one that invites students to use their values?

A major goal of values awareness lessons is to help students become aware of their values. The focus-setting question must, therefore, invite students to use their values. The ways people most frequently use their values is to make value judgments or propose a desired course of action to be implemented. Having done so, it is possible to "read back" from the value judgment or course of action to the underlying values. As a result, focus-setting questions most suitable for values awareness lessons are those that call for students to make value judgments or report a course of action.

One stem usually effective in formulating a focus-setting question that invites students to make value judgments is, *How do you feel about....?*

The stem usually effective in formulating a focus-setting question that invites students to report a course of action is, *What should be done about....?*

It should be pointed out that focus-setting questions which invite students to report a value judgment or course of action also stimulate the occurrence of other student behaviors such as reporting data, reporting predictions, generating data, reporting values, and so on in support of these value judgments or proposed courses of action. It is the natural way people respond to these kinds of focus-setting questions. On the other hand, focus-setting questions that begin with stems such as, *What happened...,* *What do you think will happen...?* usually are not suitable for values awareness. They do stimulate a discussion by inviting students to report data or make predictions. However, it is difficult to facilitate the students' awareness of their values if they are not using their values by reporting courses of action or making value judgments as a legitimate part of the discussion.

Some Other Factors to be Considered in Selecting a Focus-Setting Question

In addition to formulating or selecting topics for values awareness lessons in the light of the three criteria presented, there are some other factors which should also be taken into account. One such factor is state laws related to what teachers can and cannot do in the classroom.

Many states have laws that prohibit teachers from asking students questions about their home life, about what their parents do, or about how their parents feel about something. Many local school districts have policies in support of these kinds of state laws. Other kinds of district policies may preclude the discussion of specific topics such as premarital sex, etc., by teachers and students in the classroom and in turn is another factor to be considered.

Another factor that should influence the teacher's selection of topics or questions for values awareness lessons is whether or not the topic is related to a highly frustrating or traumatic experience of one or more of the students in the classroom. For example, while to identify a topic such as divorce may be highly relevant to a group of students because they are products of divorced parents, the trauma they may have experienced may be reason enough for the teacher to avoid that topic. On the other hand, with a capable teacher this topic may be ideal for those students.

Finally, whatever topic is identified for a values awareness lesson, it must be one that the teacher can live with; one that he or she will be able to maintain an "open" climate rather than one for which the teacher has very strong feelings. In the latter case the teacher's strong feelings may come through to the students regardless of what he or she says and thereby interfere with the lesson climate. Thus, the teacher's own values also enter into the decision about what topics are appropriate for these kinds of lessons in his or her classroom.

In reviewing these four additional factors to be considered in selecting a question for a values awareness lesson it may seem at first glance that there will be few questions suitable for the classroom that are not in conflict with one or more of these factors. Actually, nothing could be further from the truth. By wording focus-setting questions thoughtfully, many potential conflicts with state laws, such as asking students about their parents or home life, can easily be avoided. For example, in most instances where the question is posed to a group rather than directed to an individual student, it is okay to ask the students how they feel about an issue or topic rather than asking them how their parents feel about it. It is okay to ask students what they think might or should be done about a given dilemma such as the use of drugs in the community rather than asking them about what their parents have done, are doing, or should be doing.

Avoiding conflict with district policies is also relatively easily dealt with. If the school district has a policy prohibiting classroom discussion of premarital sex, do not discuss that topic. We have seen several effective values-related educational programs, teaching strategies, or classroom activities prohibited in some school districts because of a teacher's thoughtless or stubborn judgment in the selection of topics. As a result, they "lost the baby with the bath water." The place to fight existing school district policies is at a district board meeting, not in the classroom. Taking school district policies into consideration when selecting or formulating a focus-setting question merely means knowing what school district policies are, and finding ways to work legitimately within them.

The other two factors present a bit more of a challenge for the teacher. In one instance, the teacher will find it necessary to keep informed, as best he or she can, about the lives of the students. In doing so, the teacher will be better able to avoid selecting topics or issues for discussions that may be overly disturbing or embarassing to some of the students in the group. As for the final factor, the teacher's own values, it is necessary for the teacher to keep tuned into his or her own feelings, anxieties, and concerns in order to avoid subverting the objectives of the values awareness lesson. Otherwise, instead of providing an opportunity for the students to gain some insight into their own values, the lesson becomes a platform for the teacher to espouse his or her biases, attitudes, judgments, or values. And while to do so may be appropriate for some other kinds of lessons, it is "out of bounds" for a values awareness lesson.

Setting the Stage for the Focus-Setting Question

Having selected or formulated a focus-setting question in view of the criteria and factors identified, a related issue of concern to the teacher is: *In what way will the focus-setting question be presented to the students?* Obviously, there are many different ways the question may be given to the students. Ways to present a focus-setting question may range from just stating the question for the students' response, to involving them in various kinds of group activities. But, how does the teacher decide whether to initiate the lesson by the use of the focus-setting question alone or to couple the statement of the question with some kind of presentation, activity, or discussion designed to set the stage for the question?

The teacher's purpose in using some means to set the stage for a focus-setting question is to get the students geared up for, tuned in to, or otherwise motivated to respond to the discussion topic. Obviously, there are those instances in which it is not necessary for the teacher to set the stage for the discussion. For example, if the students' classroom or homeroom was vandalized and many of the students' work was destroyed or some of their property solen, there would probably be no need for the teacher to set the stage for a question such as, *How do you feel about people who destroy school property?* The vandals would have set the stage for the discussion by their action. Similarly, some spontaneous event on the school playground or campus such as a fight, disturbance, or visitation by the Tooth Fairy can set the stage for related questions.

In these kinds of situations, the teacher does not have to set the stage for the focus-setting question because it is automatically taken care of. In most other situations, however, some action by the teacher to set the stage is required in order to:

- Help the students relate their present knowledge to the specific focus-setting question; and/or
- Build the necessary knowledge related to the topic if the focus-setting question is to have meaning for the students; and/or
- Build the momentum for the values awareness lesson by developing the students' understanding of the topic before the focus-setting question is posed; and/or
- Help the students see the relevance of the focus-setting question to their lives, interests, or concerns.

It is apparent that productive focus-setting questions have their meaning for people in some kind of context. Setting the stage for the question is taking action to establish that context for the students. In some instances, natural events in the student's lives set the stage for the discussion. With most focus-setting questions appropriate for health education, however, the teacher must take some action to set the stage for the discussion question.

Using Overhead Transparencies or Study Prints to Set the Stage

Undoubtedly, there are many ways a teacher can set the stage for a focus-setting question. In the chapter entitled, "The Values Awareness Teaching Strategy: An Overview," a script of part of a values awareness lesson was given. You may recall that Ms. Pollock, the teacher, set the stage for the focus-setting question, *What should*

Gerald do? by inviting her students to discuss what they felt was happening in a transparency shown on an overhead projector. When she felt that the students understood the situation depicted and that some momentum for the discussion had been achieved, she wrote the question on the transparency. The stage was set, the focus-setting question presented, and the values awareness lesson was initiated.

The stage for this focus-setting question could also have been set in other ways as well. A study print, unfinished story, case study, film or filmstrip might have been used. Obviously, to set the stage for this particular question, the theme of any of these materials would have to deal with a boy or girl who gets a venereal disease. In the sample of Ms. Pollock's lesson, she adapted a transparency designed for another purpose to set the stage for a values awareness lesson focus-setting question. In addition to the School Health Education Study materials she drew on, there are many other educational materials that may be used as they are or they may be adapted in some way to set the stage for values awareness focus-setting questions.

Using Unfinished Stories to Set the Stage

The National Education Association has two volumes available entitled, "Unfinished Stories." Written several years ago, these stories should be adapted to the present day language of students to make them suitable. Unfinished stories take the students through some situation to that moment in which the major characters have a decision or choice to make. While the NEA Unfinished Stories are not intended to deal specifically with health issues, many do relate to health since they center on coping with emotional and social problems familiar to most students.

An Unfinished Story: What Should Gail Do?

(Adapted with permission from *Unfinished Stories for Use in the Classroom.* National Education Association, 1966.)

Gail sat alone, chewing on a dry peanut butter sandwich. It would have gone down more easily and tasted better if she'd had an orange to go with it, but according to her mother, oranges cost too much money for her family. Gail watched a group of girls by the window. They were laughing at something the boys were doing on the playground. She would have given anything to be with them, but the other girls never included her. You were "in" or you were "out," Gail decided miserably. She was obviously "out."

To be popular in school, you had to wear the kinds of clothes the other girls were wearing. Right now, the style at school was paisley "maxies." Gail not only didn't have a paisley print "maxie," she didn't have a print dress of any kind. All she had was one or two shabby skirts, a few blouses, and an old gray sweater her aunt had thrown away. Just that morning at breakfast, Gail had tried to explain to her mother how important it was for her to dress like the other girls. "You don't have to tell me how it feels not to belong," Mother had said. "I never belonged to anything in my whole life. But there is no use crying over what you haven't got. You'll have to be liked because you are a good friend and cheerful."

Gail didn't think she had much to be cheerful about. She wasn't pretty and she couldn't think of clever things to say. She didn't have any particular talent to do something special, like play a musical instrument or sing. She was sure that even if she acted cheerful every minute, she still wouldn't become one of the group of girls.

The girls were nice enough but they didn't let her in on their secrets or trade clothes with her or invite her home. Some of the other girls in the class were "out" too, but this was because they wanted it that way. Some of them were honor students who liked to spend their time studying. Gail didn't think she was smart enough to be "in" with them and she didn't think they were much fun anyway. She wanted to be part of the popular group of girls.

●   Focus-Setting Question: *What Should Gail Do?*   ●

Using Scenarios to Set the Stage

Similar to Unfinished Stories, scenarios describe a "make believe" situation or event that the students are involved in. Unfinished Stories usually end with the focus-setting question: *"What should _____ do?"* Scenarios, on the other hand, frequently conclude with the question, *"What would you do in this situation?"* While most frequently scenarios are read by the teacher or the students, some may be adapted to a script format in which students role play the various roles depicted in the scenario. These kinds of scenarios might conclude with the focus-setting question, *"What would you do next in that situation?"* Published in 1972 by the National Highway Traffic Administration and the National Institute on Alcohol Abuse and Alcoholism, "Alcohol and Alcohol Safety," a curriculum manual for the upper elementary, junior high and senior high levels, includes a number of scenarios useful to the teacher of health education.

A Scenario: The Big League Game

(Adapted from *Alcohol and Alcohol Safety, Upper Elementary,* National Highway Traffic Administration & the National Institute on Alcohol Abuse and Alcoholism, 1972.)

You are an elementary school-age boy. While playing Little League baseball, you have become friendly with Richard Smith, who is another outfielder on your team. He's really a great kid and a fantastic ball player. Sometimes he tells stories about some of the wild drinking parties his parents have had. You know from your other friends at school that Richard's father is an alcoholic, but you don't see that should have anything to do with your friendship with Richard. Actually, it makes Richard seem a little more interesting to you, especially because your father is a very quiet man. You wonder what it's like having a father who frequently gets drunk and beats up his wife.

Yesterday during the game, Richard told you his father was going to take him to a big league baseball game. Richard said it was okay with his father if you would like to go along with them. You don't usually get a chance to go to a big league game, so this was a big chance for you, and secretly you're very curious to meet Richard's father, too.

It's dinnertime now at your home, and you are seated at the dinner table with your Mom and Dad. You wonder if you should just go with Richard without telling your folks or ask them. Since your folks know Richard's dad is an alcoholic, you are concerned that they might not let you go to the ball game with him.

- Focus-Setting Question: *What would you do?* •

Using Short Stories, Literature or Magazine Articles to Set the Stage

Literature, short stories, and magazine articles can also be useful in setting the stage for a focus-setting question. In these cases, however, productive focus-setting questions most frequently are those that invite the students to make value judgments about what one or more of the characters did or said. As a result, questions such as, *"How do you feel about what _____ did?* are usually used.

A Stort Story: The Miracle Drug

(Adapted from the *Heinz Story* used by L. Kohlberg, Professor, Harvard Graduate School of Education.)

A woman was suffering from an extremely rare, painful disease. According to the most qualified doctors, there was a 95 percent chance that in three months she would become nearly completely paralyzed and would suffer a very painful bedridden existence thereafter. There was one medicine that offered a 50 percent chance of a cure.

The only medicine presently available was developed by a physician who spent several years in the research and development of the substance. Furthermore, he financed the development with his own money. For a complete treatment, the medicine cost the doctor $100. However, he charged each patient $2,000 (20 times his cost in time and ingredients) of which he donated $1,600 to an orphan's home.

The woman's concerned husband found himself without the $2,000 he needed to buy the treatment. After selling their household goods and automobile, $800 was all he could raise. His efforts to acquire loans or welfare aid proved fruitless. The husband pleaded with the physician to give him the medicine for the $800 plus the promise to pay the remaining $1,200 on installment payments. The physician rejected the offer. He said, "I developed this substance after years of financial sacrifice and because there are never more than two or three cases of this disease a year, I must demand the full amount in cash."

The husband felt desperate. His wife needed the medicine now, but there was no way he knew of to get it for her except to steal it. He turned to his minister for advice. The minister told him that stealing was against the ten commandments and that his wife's suffering was God's will and he shouldn't interfere with what God had willed. His best friend refused to advise him because he didn't want to get involved. His wife pleaded with him to steal, even murder if necessary to get the medicine.

One night, the husband broke into the doctor's office, stole the medicine his wife needed, and in a fit of anger, destroyed the remaining medicine and the formula.

- Focus-Setting Question: *Who was the most reprehensible — the woman, the husband, the physician, the minister, the friend?* •

Literature

The following are a few examples of books that may be used to set the stage for a health-related values awareness lesson.

Daly, Maureen: *The Seventeenth Summer* (Pocket Books, 1968). This is a story about the first love of a 17-year-old girl. On page 163, her older boyfriend takes her to a German restaurant where she has a coke. Her boyfriend suggests she try a stein of beer. She gives in "for fun," even though she feels it is not "ladylike." After her second beer, she becomes very talkative and laughs a lot, then becomes sleepy. Later on she feels that she had a wonderful evening. (Mature reading.)

Woody, Regina J.: *One Day At A Time* (Westminster, 1968). This story is about a 13-year-old girl whose mother is an alcoholic. Her mother eventually drinks herself unconscious and is taken to a hospital. Later the mother has a birthday party for the girl at which the mother gets drunk, to the embarassment of the girl. (Mature reading.)

Sherburne, Zoa: *Jennifer* (Morrow, 1959). A story about a girl whose mother is an alcoholic. She learns to cope with this type of family situation. (Mature reading.) (Hardbound only.)

Miller, Warren: *The Cool World* (Crest). A novel about a gang of ghetto blacks in New York City and their lives. They drink to get courage to fight other neighborhood gangs. Pages 148-155. Uses ghetto dialect. (Mature reading.)

Hinton, S.E.: *The Outsiders* (Dell, 1969). A novel written by a teenage girl about two warring juvenile gangs. Pages 49-51. A scene is described in which one gang is drunk and starts a fight with the other gang. (Average reading.)

Twain, Mark: *The Adventures of Huckleberry Finn* (Bantam). A story about a young boy's adventures on the Mississippi River in the 1880s. His father is an alcoholic. In one scene, his father gets the D.T.s. Pages 13, 19-34. (Mature reading.)

Using Group Activities to Set the Stage

It was mentioned earlier that criteria useful in selecting or formulating a focus-setting question is relevance. While various group activities such as these outlined or described by Simon et al [9] and Pfeiffer and Jones [10] may be used to set the stage for a specific discussion question, other activities are useful to enable the teacher to select the question most relevant to a group of students.

Group Activity: Forced Choice

(Adapted for upper elementary students from the activity demonstrated by Sidney Simon, Association for Supervision and Curriculum Development National Conference, St. Louis, 1969.)

For this activity, the teacher has prepared a list of phrases on a transparency that completes the stem, *How strongly do you feel about....?* A key word is underlined in each phrase. The students are given a sheet of paper that has been divided into the same number of boxes as the number of phrases to be read. The boxes are numbered in sequence.

In structuring for the activity, the teacher informs the students that a certain number of questions are to be read aloud, one at a time. Each time a question is read, they are to decide how strongly they feel about it and write the key word in the appropriate box. Be sure the students are aware that they are ranking strong feelings which may be either positive or negative versus weak feelings that may be either positive or negative. Box number one represents something they feel very strong about, number two next, and so on. The last box will represent something they don't care about very much. In other words, the students will be ranking the items they are highly concerned about toward one end of the scale and those they care little about at the other end.

When they've finished, they will have one key word in each box. The questions are read aloud, with the key word underlined on the transparency.

How strongly do you feel about:†

1. *Telling* on a friend who has done something really wrong?

2. Kids who *shoplift?*

3. Kids who *cheat* to win a game?

4. Kids who fool around with *drugs?*

5. Having *casseroles* for dinner?

6. Sharing a *bedroom* with your brother or sister?

7. Kids who eat a lot of *junk food?*

8. People who *smoke* cigarettes in restaurants?

---

†*This particular list of topics was developed for upper elementary students by Ar Stebin, Oneonta School, South Pasadena Unified School District, 1974.*

After all of the questions are read, the students are given time to make any shifts they want to.

Next, the students are organized into groups of three or more. Each group is invited to arrive at a consensus of the first three items. They are given from five to ten minutes to decide. Each of the groups then writes the key word of their No. 1, No. 2, and No. 3 rated questions horizontally on a 2″ wide strip of transparency material (Figure 11).

FIGURE 11

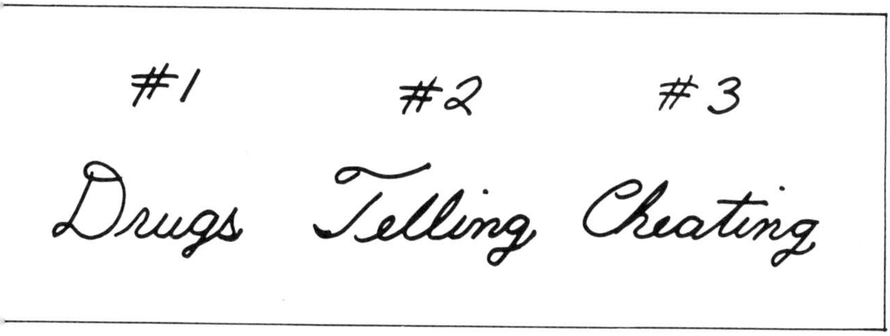

The strips from each group are then placed on an overhead projector to allow the class to see and discuss the rankings made by all of the groups.

When each group's ranking of the first three topics has been recorded on the transparency shown on the overhead, and discussed in the total group, two things have been accomplished. The teacher has information about which topics are of greatest concern or relevance to the students. Furthermore, the period of discussion in the small groups serves to get the students thinking about the topics, sharing their ideas, and listening to the ideas of others. Thus, this activity enables the teacher both to select a question relevant to the students and to get them talking and thinking about it as a way of setting the stage for the values awareness lesson to follow. The teacher then selects one of the more frequently rated top choices and poses it as a focus-setting question. For example, in one class, drugs came up as the No. 1 item in 8 out of the 12 groups. Other groups had rated it as No. 2. So the teacher used that as a focus-setting question for a Values Awareness lesson.

- Focus-Setting Question: *What should be done about kids who fool around with drugs?* •

In some cases the values awareness lesson may follow the Forced Choice Activity or the actual discussion may be initiated on the next day.

Using Films or Television Programs to Set the Stage

For years teachers have followed the use of a film or television program in the classroom with a discussion of what students saw or heard, the key points made, or what they got out of it. Used in this way, the teacher's purpose in showing the film or telecast was to introduce or present some information to begin to develop a new concept for the students. The discussion serves to highlight the specific information or concepts the students should learn. There are obviously other purposes teachers have in using films and television programs in the classroom.

Films and television programs can also be used to set the stage for a values awareness lesson. In this case, however, rather than centering the follow-up discussion on what was depicted in the program, the emphasis is on getting students to consider what they think a given character should do or how they felt about a character(s) or situation. Since most films or television programs are intended to tell a story, focus-setting questions beginning with the stem, *How do you feel about....* are usually most appropriate. Focus-setting questions beginning with the stem, *What should* ——————— *do?* may be used if the telecast or film is cut off at a critical point in the story. That is, the film or telecast is stopped just after a leading character is confronted with a decision to be made or an action to be taken.

More recently, educational film and television producers have developed programs designed to set the stage for classroom discussion. Of particular interest to health educators are the program series entitled INSIDE/OUT and SELF-INCORPORATED. Produced by the Agency For Instructional Television, Bloomington, Indiana, the programs center on an array of mental health issues related to the lives of 8- to 10-year-olds and 11- to 13-year-old children respectively.

Programs such as these that deal with "heavy" value loaded subjects provide an ideal stimulus for a values awareness lesson.

INSIDE/OUT: I Dare You

(Portions of "Inside/Out, A Guide For Teachers," page 62 reprinted with the permission of the Agency For Instructional Television, formerly National Instructional Television, Bloomington, Indiana.)

Clarissa, a new girl in the neighborhood, wants to join the "gang." To be accepted as a member, she must carry out a potentially dangerous dare. The gang is also shaken by the potential danger and debates whether the dare is necessary and how hard it should be.

In a series of flashbacks each child recounts his particular dare. Yes, Clarissa must accept the dare to join the gang; her trial will come later in the day.

Torn between a desire for social acceptance and a concern for her safety, Clarissa fantasizes many of the possible consequences of taking the dare and argues with herself about whether membership in the group is worth the risk.

When the moment of decision arrives, she is urged on by the gang, who shout fiercely, "Go! Go! Go!" As the tension reaches its highest point the program ends.... What has Clarissa decided to do?

• Focus-Setting Question: *What Should Clarissa Do? Or, How do you feel about kids who try to make their friends take a dare?* •

Using Current Events to Set the Stage

Perhaps one of the best sources of current topics of concern in the local community, city, state, nations, or world is the newspaper. Some newspapers even present positions for and against current topics to stimulate the reader's thinking. While reading current events in elementary classes, health, civics, or social science classes is a common occurrence, it is probably fair to assume that in few instances are such newspaper articles used to set the stage for a values awareness lesson.

One shortcoming in using newspaper articles is that though related to health education, a specific article may not present a topic of interest to the students. And the best topics are those for which the students hold differing points of view or about which they hold strong feelings. One way to check out the student's interest in and reaction to an article is to use the "What Do You Think?" approach. In this case the teacher (or students) select two or more health-related newspaper articles. Each article is taped to the center of a larger piece of chart paper with the heading, "What Do You Think?" (Figure 12).

Over the period of one or more days the students are invited to write their responses to an article on the chart paper. They may be initiated if the students are willing to do so.

Those newspaper articles that stimulate response, that represent very strong feelings, or that represent divergent points of view usually offer good topics for a values awareness lesson. In addition to helping the teacher identify a topic of interest to the students, the current events approach gets the students thinking and talking about the topic before the actual values awareness lesson is initiated.

FIGURE 12

What Do You Think?

Please write your reactions here on this bulletin board. Add your name or initials to your comment.

Nursing Home Owner
Convicted

The first trial of a criminal case filed by City Atty. Burt Pines' special nursing home unit ended Thursday with a conviction of Dora Friedlander, who was accused of allowing board and care patients to become infested with lice.

As owner-operator of Commonwealth Manor in Los Angeles, she was found guilty of five misdemeanor counts by Municipal Judge Dickran Tevrizian. Her sentencing is scheduled for May 27.

The conviction included three counts of willfully failing to provide assistance necessary for the daily activities of the nursing home residents.

Another count charged that patients' clothes and food trays were dirty and unsanitary. The final count alleged that the owner-operator allowed a patient to be in charge of the facility in her absence.

LA Times, April 30, 1976

Disgusting!
R.C.

I'd never put my folks in a nursing home.
W.F.

Some people will do anything for money
Bus

How could anyone be so inhuman?
Edith

This is another example of the failure of state licensing boards to enforce rules and regulations!
Jodi Hoffman

She sounds sicker than the people she's supposed to be taking care of!
J.T.

That's the height of irresponsibility
Jane

It's time we all take a good look at the problem. It's a disgrace on the national level
Shirley P.

How could anyone do something like that and live with themselves?
Pat N.

Obviously the various techniques discussed in this chapter are only illustrative of many different ways a teacher might set the stage for a values awareness lesson. Other ways might be to take a field trip, view a film strip, invite a speaker to talk to the students, stage a debate, and so on. Rather than identify one of these techniques as best, the most effective approach is to use a variety of ways to set the stage for a values awareness lesson over the course of the semester. It is important to note, however, that:

a film is only a film,

a picture is only a picture,

a story is only a story, and

an activity is only an activity.

Whether any of these techniques is to become a values awareness lesson depends on what the teacher does and does not do.

12

Characteristic Student Behaviors Related to the Values Awareness Teaching Strategy

Helping students learn to communicate effectively and to develop their ability to explicate their own values does not "just happen" in the classroom. Achieving these ends with students requires several teacher competencies. One of these competencies is the ability to recognize what it is the students are doing as they participate in such lessons. What the students do is a base from which the teacher decides what he or she might do, can do, or should do next.

Seven voluntarily initiated student behaviors related to the Values Awareness Teaching Strategy have been identified. They are:
- Focus Setting.
- Reporting Course of Action.
- Reporting Value Judgment.
- Reporting Value.
- Reporting Prediction.
- Reporting Data.
- Generating Data.

On the pages which follow, each of these student behaviors is described in detail and a few examples of each are provided. We note that these student behaviors are not discussed here because they are what we want students to do as they participate in a values awareness lesson. Rather, these are ways students naturally respond.

A Description of the Voluntarily Initiated Student Behaviors

Focus Setting

Focus Setting is the act of recognizing, selecting, or identifying a topic or issue for discussion. This student behavior includes those instances in which the student: (1) presents a new topic of his own; (2)

revises or restates a topic presented by the teacher or another student;
(3) selects a topic for discussion from among alternatives; (4) indicates
when he feels another student has unannouncedly shifted to a new
topic; or (5) questions another student to determine if the other
student has shifted to a new topic.

STUDENT: *Today, can we talk about whether or not kids in high
school should be allowed to marry if they want to?*

STUDENT: *To me it's not racism we should be talking about.
We need to discuss how we can eliminate poverty and give
equal treatment to minorities.*

STUDENT: *Of all those topics listed, I'd like to discuss the one
about the effects of pollution on our health; what should the
government do to protect the people from industrial air
pollution?*

STUDENT: *Hey, wait a minute Gus, what you just said — you're
talking about whether it's good or bad to take a dare and we're
talking about how we feel about people who try to get you to
take a dare.*

STUDENT: *Jan, when you said you thought that child molesters
should be severely punished, weren't you talking about another
issue?*

Reporting Course of Action

Reporting A Course of Action is the act of stating what might be
done relative to a given topic. The emphasis is on proposing some
action to be taken. Usually as people report a course of action they do
so because it seems to be a viable alternative to them. The course of
action therefore carries an implicit value judgment about it.

STUDENT: *One thing might be to make sure that all elderly
people get at least one warm meal a day.*

STUDENT: *An alternative is to provide everyone with free
immunizations.*

STUDENT: *We should teach kids to respect drugs when they're
young rather than passing laws about what you can and can't
buy.*

More sophisticated Reporting Course of Action student behaviors
include some specification of the circumstances or conditions under
which the course of action reported would be most appropriate or

effective. Reporting Course of Action with Conditions is recorded RCAC.

STUDENT: *If he has a good relationship with Manual he should tell him that he really didn't mean to put the Chicanos down. If he doesn't have a good relationship with him, then it's probably better not to say anything.*

Reporting Value Judgment

Reporting a Value Judgment is the act of presenting a statement intended to communicate that the speaker feels something is good or bad. All value judgments include two elements; one that specifies worth (or lack of worth), and another element that relates that specification of worth to something. *The food was superb.* The word "superb" specifies worth, and, "superb" was related to "the food."

People may specify worth (or lack of worth) by using swear words (Oh pshaw!); colloquialisms (It's going to the dogs); value words (He's an honest fellow); polar words (great/awful); a rhetorical question (You really think that?); trigger words (Un-American); gross over-statements (Everyone will end up using pot); or, reporting a physiological or psychological state (I'm very upset about...). People may make value judgments about their own behavior, the behavior of others, an object, event, idea, a particular person or people in general, a condition, place, institution, prediction, course of action, judgment, etc. In other words, people may make a value judgment about anything!

It should be noted that in the context of actual dialogue the relating element may be implicit rather than explicit. For example, *I agree with Philomena* is intended to mean, *I agree with Philomena's suggestion.*

STUDENT: *I like fresh fruit in the summertime.*

STUDENT: *You really are a warm human being, Val.*

STUDENT: *I don't like compulsory immunization as the way to fight communicable diseases.*

STUDENT: *Anyone who tries to jive me because I'm black is a phoney.*

STUDENT: *That's a great idea.*

More sophisticated RVJ student behaviors may include the specification of circumstances or conditions when the value judgment would be most relevant. Reporting a Value Judgment with conditions is recorded RVJC.

Reporting Value

Reporting A Value is the act of making a value statement about one's own values or about the values of someone else, an institution, a group of people, etc. The Reporting Value student behavior includes three elements. One element specifies the value, another labels the value as such, and the third relates the value to something. Values are usually expressed in positive terms.

The Reporting Value student behavior seldom occurs until students have participated in several Values Awareness Lessons in which the teacher has used the Inferring Values Dialogue on several occasions.

STUDENT: *Friendliness is one of my values when it comes to choosing a physician.*

STUDENT: *One of my values about drug treatment programs is that they are readily available to those who wish to use them.*

STUDENT: *From what I heard Yoshi say, Mrs. Lopez, I think that one of her values about teachers is that they treat boys and girls the same.*

In many instances the Reporting Value student behavior first occurs in a less complete form. In this case, the student specifies some general class of human experience and specifies a characteristic deemed desirable about that class, but he fails to label the characteristic cited as a value. In other words, at this point he is becoming aware of what is important to him, but does not yet label it as a value.

STUDENT: *Friendliness is important to me when it comes to choosing a physician.*

STUDENT: *Hector, it looks like what's really important to you about teachers is that they treat boys and girls the same.*

Reporting Prediction

Reporting a Prediction is the act of forecasting outcomes which may result from implementing a course of action. The Reporting Prediction student behavior is often cited as a rationale for a Course of Action or a Value Judgment, or for holding a particular value.

STUDENT: *I know what's going to happen if you do away with the dress code in school; there will be an increase in disciplinary problems.*

STUDENT: *If we don't do something about the syphilis problem, we're going to have a lot of people who will go blind and insane.*

STUDENT: *Sure, then you'll end up hiring women because they're women instead of because they can do the job.*

Reporting Data

Reporting data is the act of stating either (1) nonjudgmental characteristics of a person, place, event, institution, object; (2) observable human behavior; (3) nonjudgmental descriptions of conditions of some place, object, institution, event, person, or, the psychological or physiological state of an individual. Reporting data is making a data statement. The student may cite data as his rationale for a Course of Action reported or a Value Judgment he made. Validity or accuracy of the data reported are not criteria considered in classifying a student behavior as Reporting Data.

STUDENT: *Farnsworth told me he got impetigo from smoking marijuana.*

STUDENT: *I heard that you can get some kinds of VD from door knobs.*

STUDENT: *A methadone maintenance program is one legal way that people who are dependent on heroin can meet that psychological need.*

STUDENT: *Would you look at that, one of Frieda's eyes is crossed!*

STUDENT: *I sure feel lousy.*

STUDENT: *I ate lunch in the cafeteria today and I feel sick.*

Generating Data

Generating Data is the act of making a statement about specific data the student needs or wants or actually taking action to generate the data.

STUDENT: *I need to know what happens to people who have syphilis and don't get treatment for it.*

STUDENT: *I need some information about where all the free clinics in our community are located and what they do.*

STUDENT: *Just how does the fluoride in toothpaste work to prevent cavities?*

Additional Student Behaviors

The most critical behaviors students use as they are engaged in a values awareness lesson have been discussed earlier in this chapter. There are, however, other kinds of things students do as a natural product of a discussion that are highly relevant to values awareness. For example, like teachers, and perhaps as an outgrowth of observing the teacher working with them, students begin using a Clarifying behavior when they do not understand and an Acknowledging behavior when they do understand.

In addition to Clarifying and Acknowledging behaviors, all of the student behaviors discussed earlier have one thing in common; they are voluntarily initiated. That is, the teacher did not call on the students or otherwise prompt them to report a course of action, make a value judgment, report data, and so on. There are other things students do as a response to questions directed to them by the teacher or by other students during the course of a discussion.

To provide a way of identifying what students do in response to the Clarifying and certain Values Awareness Teaching Strategies Goal Directed and Diagnostic teaching behaviors, a relatively simple technique has been used very effectively. The technique uses the name of the teaching behavior with a Y, N, or S added. The letter "Y" means the student responded consistent with the intent of the teaching behavior; yes, the teaching behavior worked. "N" means the student responded, but that response was inconsistent with what the teaching behavior called for; no, the teaching behavior did not work. "S" means that the student was silent in response to the teaching behavior. For example, when the teacher uses a Clarifying teaching behavior (CL) and the student responds by restating, rephrasing, adding to what he or she said or defining a term he or she used, the student's response is identified as CLY; Clarifying, yes! If, on the other hand, the student responds by changing the subject, the response is identified as CLN; Clarifying, no. This means that the Clarifying teaching behavior did not have the intended effect.

Finally, if the teacher uses a Clarifying teaching behavior and the student looks confused or otherwise unable to respond, and does not, the student's response is identified as CLS — Clarifying Silence. Of course, whenever the student responds to a Clarifying, Inferring Value, or any of the probe teaching behaviors with silence, the teacher would want to relieve any pressure the student may feel to respond by using a Structuring teaching behavior such as, *That's ok, Ben, you don't have to respond right now. You can think about it if you'd like to.*

As a result of using this Y, N, S approach, Figure 13 is a list of additional student behaviors that may be easily identified.

FIGURE 13

Preceding Teaching Behavior	Student's Response		
	Yes	No	Silence
Clarifying	CLY	CLN	CLS
Probe for Rationale	PRY	PRN	PRS
Probe for Data	PDY	PDN	PDS
Probe for Data Source	PDSY	PDSN	PDSS
Inferring Value	IVY	IVN	IVS
Probe for Process Awareness	PPAY	PPAN	PPAS
Probe for Conditions	PCY	PCN	PCS
Probe for Values	PVY	PVN	PVS

There are two advantages in using the Y, N, and S approach to identifying student's responses to Clarifying, Inferring Values, and the probe teaching behaviors. The first is that when plotted on a *"T" System Lesson Analysis Form,* discussed in the chapter on evaluation, the effect of the probe teaching behaviors can be readily assessed. "Y" means they are working, "N" or "S" means they are not. A second advantage of this approach is that it enables the teacher to easily differentiate between those behaviors students initiate of their own volition, such as Focus Setting, Reporting Course of Action, Reporting Value Judgment and so on, from those that are in response to the teacher probes. A simple count of the range and frequency of student behaviors used during a lesson or an analysis of a "T" System of the lesson therefore makes it possible for the teacher to study the relationship between what students do that is self-initiated and what they do that is in response to a direct question from the teacher.

Identifying Student Behavior

When teachers observe students discussing a topic or issue, the students frequently make statements that can be classified as a series of different student behaviors. For example:

STUDENT: *I think teenagers shouldn't be allowed to smoke because they'll probably get lung cancer more easily.*

This student behavior may be classified as two behaviors:

STUDENT: *I think teenagers shouldn't be allowed to smoke...*(Reporting Course of Action)*...because they'll probably get lung cancer more easily.* (Reporting Prediction) Thus, this statement would be classified as Reporting Course of Action — Reporting Prediction.

On the other hand, classifying a student's statement into its component parts may become unmanageable in many situations. Instead the teacher may prefer to identify only the primary message communicated. Because the student's primary message in the example provided earlier appears to be to communicate a preferred course of action among several proposed, it would be classified as Reporting Course of Action.

Which way should you classify student behavior? You decide. In some situations listening for one primary message communicated will suffice. In other occasions, however, it may be important to attend to the various component parts of the student's behavior.

13

Using the Values Awareness
Teaching Behaviors

One aspect of the successful implementation of the Values Awareness Teaching Strategy is knowing what to do to create the classroom climate for values awareness, knowing what to do to facilitate the student's growth toward the goals for values awareness and knowing what to do to generate diagnostic data about the student's growth. But knowing what to do, that is, knowing what the teaching behaviors are, is not enough. Another aspect of the successful implementation of the Values Awareness Teaching Strategy is knowing when to use these teaching behaviors. What follows are guidelines that are helpful to determine which teaching behavior is most appropriate at the time. Since this teaching strategy is responsive in nature, it is what the student does that suggests the alternatives open to the teacher. We underscore that the interaction alternatives to be discussed are intended to serve as guidelines. Teacher judgment based on who the student is and what he or she has done in the past should influence both the teacher's decisions about what teaching behavior should be used as well as the specific words chosen to implement that teaching behavior.

Guidelines for Using the Basic Teaching Behaviors

To initiate the lesson, the Structuring teaching behavior is used to inform the students about how they will be working, what they can expect of their teacher, and what the teacher expects of them. The Focus Setting teaching behavior is used to inform the students about the specific question or issue for discussion.

TEACHER: *In our discussion today, let's work as we did last week, remember?...* (Structuring) *The question I'd like to invite you to respond to is, "What do you think the boy in this picture should do when the girl he really likes comes up and offers him a drink of vodka?"* (Focus Setting)

Having initiated the lesson by establishing the lesson structure and specifying the topic for discussion, it is the students' turn to begin the discussion. If they do not do so, the teacher uses Teacher Silence to communicate that, unlike many other lessons, a values awareness lesson rests on voluntary student participation. If they have nothing to say, nothing will be said.

While the Structuring teaching behavior is used to initiate the lesson, it is also used during the lesson where the teacher feels it is necessary to add to or change the lesson structure, or when he or she must take some action to maintain the lesson structure. This may be necessary if there is structure breakdown; various members of the group begin talking to each other or when one student makes a derogatory remark about another student. If the teacher or a classmate poses a question to another student and the teacher senses the student is unable or unwilling to respond, a Structuring teaching behavior is used to maintain the lesson structure by relieving the psychological pressure to respond. If the student attempts to generate data and the teacher identifies a data source he may use, the teacher may also use a Structuring teaching behavior to maintain the lesson structure by reminding the student that it is up to her or him to get that data if he or she wants it.

As students participate in the lesson, there are those occasions when the teacher does not understand what the student is saying or when he or she is unsure of the specific behavior being utilized (e.g., whether the student is Reporting Data or Making a Value Judgment). A Clarifying teaching behavior may be utilized. Of course, when a student is talking to the teacher and the teacher does understand, an Acknowledging teaching behavior should be used. On those occasions when the students want to generate some data they feel they need in relation to the discussion question, the teacher uses a Responding to Student's Data Generating teaching behavior as he or she takes some action to make it possible for the student to get that data.

From time to time, as values awareness lessons unfold, students may knowingly or unknowingly shift from the original topic of discussion. To maintain the integrity of the lesson, it is incumbent on the teacher to help students recognize this shift. At the same time, it is also incumbent on the teacher to let the group know if they are to make a shift to the "new" topic or if they are to continue with the topic stated at the outset of the lesson. To alert the students to the shift in the discussion topic, the Focus Setting teaching behavior is used. This teaching behavior is followed with a Structuring teaching behavior in order to let the group know that: (1) they should shift to the new topic; (2) they should continue with the original topic for now and discuss the new one later; (3) they will be unable to discuss the "new" topic in the classroom; or (4) they are to decide whether to discuss it or not.

The following are some examples of the use of the Focus Setting and Structuring teaching behavior in combination.

STUDENT: During a discussion about alcohol, Kenton states, *I think that we should talk about sex, like going to bed with girls. That's what we should be talking about instead of drinking.* (Focus Setting)

In some school districts, the topic of premarital sex is against school policies, so the topic proposed by the student in the above example would automatically be out-of-bounds for the classroom. The Focus Setting teaching behavior is used to label the new topic and Structuring is used to rule it out for the classroom.

TEACHER: *You've raised another topic for discussion, Kenton.* (Focus Setting) *However, present school policies don't permit classroom discussion about that kind of a topic, so we'll have to pass on it.* (Structuring)

In some school districts, the topic of premarital sex is not against school policies, so the topic may be okay. However, it may be that the teacher would feel uncomfortable about it or would be unable to deal with it effectively. In this case, the Structuring teaching behavior might be:

TEACHER: *You've raised another topic for discussion, Kenton.* (Focus Setting) *However, I wouldn't feel comfortable in dealing with that topic right now, so we'll have to pass on it for now. Perhaps later on in the semester.* (Structuring)

In some instances where the topic of premarital sex is not against school policies, the teacher may decide to structure the new topic out for now because of the intense involvement of the students in the present topic of discussion, or he or she may want to let the students decide if it is a topic they would like to discuss.

TEACHER: *You've raised another topic for discussion, Kenton.* (Focus Setting) *However, because we are deeply involved in another topic right now, I'll make note of that one on the board for now. Perhaps we can: (1) discuss it next time,* (depending upon the student's interest) (Structuring) *(2) let the group decide if they want to deal with it next time.* (Structuring)

In each of the few foregoing examples, the Focus Setting and Structuring teaching behaviors were used in response to a given student behavior. Yet, each Structuring teaching behavior came out with a different message depending on school policies, the teacher's ability to deal with the topic, the teacher's appraisal of the students' ability to deal with the topic, the teacher's appraisal of the students' interest in the topic, or the teacher's recognition of an opportunity to let the students decide for themselves (because it was within school policies and the teacher felt he or she could deal with it and the students would be able to deal with the topic in a mature way).

Figure 14 visually summarizes the relationship between what students do in a values awareness lesson and the teacher's use of the Basic Teaching Behaviors.

Summarized in another way, as teacher, Clarify when you do not understand what a student is saying or doing, Acknowledge when you do. Use Focus Setting to help students become aware of when they shift discussion topics, Respond to Student's Data Generating when they want to generate data, and use the Structuring teaching behavior as necessary to maintain the lesson climate and integrity. And when the students are silent, so is the teacher.

FIGURE 14

Student Behavior	Basic Teaching Behaviors	
Focus Setting	(CL)* STR, FS	
Reporting Course of Action		FS - Focus Setting
Reporting Value Judgment		CL - Clarifying
		STR - Structuring
Reporting Value	– (CL, STR) A	A - Acknowledging
Reporting Prediction		RDG - Responding to Student's Data Generating
Reporting Data		
Generating Data	(A, CL, STR) RDG	TS - Teaching Silence
Student Silence	TS	

*Behaviors in parentheses are used as necessary. Those outside of parenthesis are essential to maintain the climate of a values awareness lesson.

Guidelines for Using the Values Awareness Goal-Directed Teaching Behaviors

Some take the position that student dialogue alone facilitates values awareness. *Just give them an opportunity to discuss health-related issues and good things will happen.* However, even though students talk to each other while they are in and out of school, few are actually aware of their values, much less know what a value is. While we recognize that lessons have been heralded in which the teacher got the discussion started and the students would keep things going on their own, we feel the teacher has a more critical job to do than just sit and listen. This is particularly so when values awareness is the goal for instruction at the time. It is our position that if values awareness is to be an outcome of health education, the teacher must be willing and able to utilize the Values Awareness Goal-Directed teaching behaviors to yield this outcome with his or her students. Before the use of these teaching behaviors is discussed, however, it is important to note that in one sense they are all interventions. That is, they are actions the teacher takes deliberately to help the students move toward the lesson goals.

In order to help the students become aware of the various behaviors they utilize during a values-related discussion, the teacher uses the Tuning In To Process teaching behavior. It is used when the students either report a course of action, report a value judgment, report a value, report a prediction, report data, or generate data. The teacher simply, and almost incidentally, labels what they have done. Certainly, the teacher does not label everything each student does as they participate in the discussion. Furthermore, as students begin giving evidence that they are aware of the various behaviors they and other students use by using that terminology as part of their incidental vocabulary, the teacher will no longer need to use this teaching behavior with those students.

When the students report a course of action or a prediction, the Probe for Data teaching behavior may be used to help students become aware of the role of data in their decision making. When students report data or seek to generate data, a Probe for Data Source may be used to help them consider the source of data as one way to assess the validity of the data.

To help students become aware of and learn to consider possible consequences or outcomes of a course of action proposed or set of values to be implemented, the Probe for Prediction teaching behavior is used. Finally, both to help students develop a concept of value and to help them become aware of their values, the Probe for Rationale and Inferring Values teaching behaviors are used in the context of an Inferring Values Dialogue when students use their values by reporting a course of action or make a value judgment.

Figure 15 visually summarizes the relationship between what students do in a values awareness lesson and the teacher's use of the Values Awareness Goal Directed teaching behaviors:

When concerned about facilitating student's growth toward the goals of values awareness lessons, the teacher is confronted with a dilemma. To sit and listen to a discussion among the students without utilizing these teaching behaviors is to forfeit the goals for values awareness lessons. On the other hand, to use these teaching behaviors without regard for the integrity of the discussion could easily disrupt the lesson flow. It is clear, therefore, that these teaching behaviors must be used thoughtfully with special regard for their effect both on the individual students within the group and on the group as a whole.

FIGURE 15

Student Behavior	VATS Goal Directed Teaching Behaviors
Focus Setting	
Reporting Course of Action	TIP, PR, IV, PD, PP
Reporting Value Judgment	TIP, PR, IV
Reporting Value	PP
Reporting Prediction	TIP, PD
Reporting Data	TIP, PDS
Generating Data	TIP, PDS

TIP - Tuning In To Process
PR - Probe for Rationale
PD - Probe for Data
PDS - Probe for Data Source
IV - Inferring Value
PP - Probe for Prediction

Guidelines for Using the Values Awareness Diagnostic Teaching Behaviors

The Basic Teaching Behaviors are used when the teacher feels it is necessary to take action to establish and maintain the lesson climate or the integrity of the discussion. The Values Awareness Goal Directed teaching behaviors are used in relation to what a student is doing at the time and what the teacher is trying to accomplish with him or her. The Values Awareness Diagnostic teaching behaviors offer one way for the teacher to assess the growth of the students toward the goals of values awareness. Obviously, these teaching behaviors are used only in those instances when the evidence of growth does not occur naturally as a normal part of the discussion.

One kind of evidence the teacher seeks about student growth is their awareness of the various behaviors they or others use during a values-loaded discussion such as: Reporting a Course of Action, Reporting a Value Judgment, Reporting a Value, Reporting a Prediction, Reporting Data or Generating Data, or when they shift the focus of the discussion. If students have not done so on their own, the teacher may use a Probe for Process Awareness teaching behavior when any one of these behaviors is used to ascertain if the students are aware of such behaviors.

Another kind of evidence of growth the teacher seeks is that the students have developed the ability to explicate and account for the conditions or circumstances that influence a course of action they propose to implement or value judgments or predictions they make. If the students have not done so on their own, the teacher may use a Probe for Conditions teaching behavior to determine if the students have indeed considered such factors.

Finally, since a central thrust of the Values Awareness Teaching Strategy is to help students conceptualize "value," to develop their ability to explicate their own values and to be able to more systematically infer the values of others, evidence of growth toward these ends is the degree to which students are able to do so. If they have not found the occasion to report their own value as a rationale for a course of action or value judgment, or if they have not otherwise given evidence of the ability to effectively infer the values of others, the Probe for Values teaching behavior may be used.

Figure 16 visually summarizes the relationship between what students do in a values awareness lesson and the teacher's use of the Values Awareness Diagnostic teaching behaviors.

The use of the Values Awareness Diagnostic teaching behaviors has been emphasized as a way of finding out about an individual student's progress toward values awareness lesson goals. These teaching behaviors are correctly used when the teacher is relatively certain that the student will be able to respond appropriately. To use them prematurely may only convince a student that he or she is unable to participate effectively in the discussion and could possibly lead to the eventual withdrawal as a participating member of the group.

In reviewing Figure 16, you will note that the Probe for Feelings teaching behavior is not included. This teaching behavior is always

FIGURE 16

Student Behavior	VATS Diagnostic Teaching Behaviors
Focus Setting	PPA
Reporting Course of Action	PPA, PC, PV
Reporting Value Judgment	PPA, PC, PV
Reporting Value	PPA
Reporting Prediction	PPA, PC
Reporting Data	PPA
Generating Data	PPA

PPA - Probe for Process Awareness
PC - Probe for Conditions
PV - Probe for Values

directed to the group as a whole so no individual student feels pressured to respond. It offers affective feedback about the lesson in general rather than information about individual student growth toward specific values awareness lesson goals. Finally, the Probe for Feelings teaching behavior is only used during the Process Dialogue after the discussion about the topic has concluded.

14

Evaluating a Values Awareness Lesson

Most teachers have a number of ways of judging the effectiveness of their teaching. Some watch their student's faces as they respond to the lesson. Some teachers direct their attention to how the students act toward each other. Some attend primarily to what the students do and say during class. Some base their judgments on what their students do at test time. Some observe for student involvement in class activities. And some use a combination of these kinds of techniques.

While all of these approaches are also useful in making judgments about the students' participation in a values awareness lesson, they only provide indirect feedback for the teacher about the effect of what he or she did during the lesson. What is also needed is a way of generating more direct feedback.

Preparing a "T" System Lesson Analysis Record of a Values Awareness Lesson

Because the Values Awareness Teaching Strategy is founded on specific identifiable student and teaching behaviors, the task of generating direct feedback about the lesson for the teacher is much easier than it is with many other teaching strategies. To do so, a "T" System Lesson Analysis Record is made. A "T" System Lesson Analysis Record is a technique used to record and organize data about student and teaching behavior which occurred during a values awareness lesson. The student and teaching behaviors are either noted on the form by an observer in the classroom during the lesson, or it may be done by the teacher through analyzing a video or audio tape recording of the lesson.

The "T" System Analysis Form looks like a capital letter "T" drawn down the center of a piece of paper. The left column is entitled, "Student" and is used to record the student behavior that occurred during the lesson. The right column is entitled, "Teacher" and is used to record teaching behavior that occurred during the lesson. The lines on a "T" System Lesson Analysis Record are numbered to facilitate ease in recording.

Data about the lesson are recorded on the "T" System Lesson Analysis Record according to the following rules:

Beginning a "T" System Lesson Analysis

The first behavior is recorded on the first line in the appropriate column. Usually the Structuring and Focus Setting teacher behaviors are used to initiate the lesson.

Student	Teacher
1.	STR-FS

Adding Behaviors

Each time a student speaks, his or her behavior is coded on a new line in the column. "Time" is defined as that period which begins when a specific student speaks and ends when someone else speaks. For example, when a student makes a comment to which the teacher or another student responds, that first student's comment is regarded as one "time."

Student	Teacher
2. RCA	

Any teaching behavior(s) that follows a given student behavior and is in direct response to that student is recorded on the same line as the student behavior, but in the "Teacher" column.

	Student	Teacher
2.	RCA	A

In those instances at the beginning or during a lesson in which the teacher directs his or her comments to the entire group, the student column is left blank and the entry is made in the teacher column.

Use of the Hyphen for Multiple Behaviors

When more than one student or teaching behavior occurs at one "time," those behaviors are separated with a hypen. If there are too many behaviors to be recorded in a column on one line, they may be recorded on the line below. A hyphen should precede the first behavior on the continued line to mark the continuation.

	Student	Teacher
3.	RCA-RP	A
4.	RVJ-RD	
5.	- RCA	STR-A

Adding Student's Names

Each "time" a different student speaks, the student's name may be written on the line next to the number. If the student cannot be recognized, a check mark may be used instead of the student's name to indicate a different student is speaking.

	Student		Teacher
3.	Francis	RCA-RP	A
4.	Bertha	RVJ-RD	
5.		-RCA	STR-A
6.	Jamie	RD	A

YN, N or S Student Behaviors for Coding Student Responses to Specific Teaching Behaviors

Some teaching behaviors, such as Clarifying, Inferring value and the Probe teaching behaviors invite a student response. As a way of recording the student's responses, the symbol of the teaching behavior plus Y, N, or S is recorded in the student column.

Y = Yes.
The student response was consistent with the intent of the teaching behavior.

N = No.
The student response was different from the intent of the teaching behavior.

S = Silence.
The student made no overt response to the teaching behavior.

	Student		Teacher
7.	Ron	RCA	CL
8.		CLY	PR
9.		PRY	A

Student's Response to TIP Teaching Behavior

Frequently, when the teacher uses a Tuning In To Process teaching behavior, students respond to it as though the teacher had used a Clarifying teaching behavior. When students respond to the Tuning In To Process by saying something like, *Yeah, that's what I said,* or by restating, rephrasing or adding more to what they said earlier, their response is identified as CLY.

	Student		Teacher
10.	Ray	RCA	TIP
11.		CLY	A

Shifting Discussion Topics

When a student starts talking about a new topic without specifying it is a new topic, that shift in topic is recorded by adding FS in parentheses after the student behavior on the same line. No hyphen is used in this case.

Student		Teacher
12. Cleo	RCA (FS)	FS-STR

"Other" Behaviors

In those instances in which there is no behavior symbol to record a given student or teaching behavior, "O" for OTHER may be used. OTHER teaching behaviors that are judged inconsistent with the Values Awareness Teaching Strategy such as making judgments about student's ideas, summarizing, using sarcasm, calling on students to get them to contribute to the discussion, and so on, can be noted by putting a slash through the "O" as shown on the teacher column below.

Student		Teacher
13. Cassy	O	A
14. Jim	RCA	A - Ø

Structure Breakdown

In those instances in which there is an apparent breakdown in the lesson structure, such as when several students begin talking at the same time, this event can be recorded in the student column with the symbol, "STRB." Of course, when the teacher responds to the structure breakdown, STR is recorded in the teacher column on the same line.

Student		Teacher
15.	STRB	STR

An Illustrative "T" System Lesson Analysis Record

In order to illustrate what a lesson looks like when recorded as a "T" System Lesson Analysis Record, we have reprinted the script from the values awareness lesson given in *"Values Awareness Teaching Strategy: An Overview."* This time, however, each of the specific student and teaching behaviors utilized during the lesson has been identified. Then, the way those behaviors are recorded on a "T" System Lesson Analysis Record is shown in the right margin.

1. MS. POLLOCK: *What I would like to do is to invite you to think about a particular issue. I'm going to present this issue to you in the form of a transparency. As we work, I want you to feel that you can share what you think should happen or ought to happen. I want you to feel comfortable in discussing the situation as you see it.*

You can share your own opinion about it or you can agree or disagree with other people's ideas or opinions. If you want some information, you can ask me and I'll try to give you the information you want, if I have it. Also, let's have one person talk at a time so we can hear what each person has to say.

I'm not going to call on anyone during the discussion. If you have something you want to say, it's up to you to make your comment. Raise your hand or just speak out if there's a moment of silence. Also, I'm not going to act as an amplifier for the group. If someone speaks and you can't hear or if you couldn't understand what they are saying, it will be up to you to let them know.

And I'm not going to make any judgments about anyone's comments by saying things like, "Good idea," or "You're right," and so on. (Structuring)

Okay, let's begin. Can you tell me what's going on here; what do you see happening? (Inviting the students to discuss a situation shown on an overhead projection screen. (Other — Setting the Stage for the Discussion Question)

JOE: *Well, that guy got kind of busted for gonorrhea and he's wondering what he should do about it.*

MS. POLLOCK: *Okay.*

ED: *Well, I don't think he's being busted. They just discovered that he had it, and I bet he's trying to decide what to do about it.*

MS. POLLOCK: *Then you're saying that he's just found out that he has it and he's trying to figure out what he should do?*

ED: *Yes.*

JIM: *He's probably also afraid that his friends will find out that he has it and what might happen to him.*

MS. POLLOCK: *All right. It's kind of the way it seems, would you agree?*

STUDENTS: Several nod in apparent agreement.

MS. POLLOCK: *Okay, then, here's the situation. Gerald is down at the Midtown Clinic and the doctor is telling him, "You've got gonorrhea."*

	Student	Teacher
1.		STR - O - FS
2.	GD	CL
3.	CLY	RDG
4.	RCA	A
5.	RCA	
6.	RVJ-RD-RP	

1. *Here's a question I'd like to invite you to respond to; "What do you think Gerald should do?"* (Focus Setting)

2. JIM: *I'm wondering if the doctor is going to tell his mom and dad.* (Generating Data)

   MS. POLLOCK: *Are you asking me if the doctor has to tell his parents?* (Clarifying)

3. JIM: *Yeah, if he has to tell them.* (Clarifying — Yes)

   MS. POLLOCK: *No. According to the California law right now, the doctor does not have to report to the parents of a minor when he or she has a venereal disease — syphilis or gonorrhea.* (Responding to Student's Data Generating)

4. JIM: *Then I think that Gerald guy should get the treatment. Right away!* (Reporting Course of Action)

   MS. POLLOCK: *Okay.* (Acknowledging)

5. ALETA: *But that's not all. He should also tell the girl he was with. She ought to know about it too.* (Reporting Course of Action)

6. JAN: *I agree.* (Reporting Value Judgment) *She could have it and not know it* (Reporting Data) *and that could mess her up, but good.* (Reporting Prediction)

7. JACK: *Right.* (Reporting Value Judgment) *She could have given it to him or he might have given it to her.* (Reporting Data)

	Student	Teacher
7.	RVJ-RD	A
8.	RP	
9.	STRB	STR
10.	RD	CL
11.	CLY	A-TIP
12.	CLY	A
13.	RCA	

MS. POLLOCK: *I see.* (Acknowledging)

8. DAPHNE: *Just think of all the girls Gerald could infect if he doesn't get treated, and...* (Reporting Value Judgment)

9. STUDENTS: Several students in the group laugh and begin commenting privately to each other about Daphne's comment. (Other — Structure Breakdown)

MS. POLLOCK: *Wait a minute people, let's give Daphne a chance to finish what she has to say.* (Structuring)

10. DAPHNE: *Well I just wanted to say that it can give him lots of other trouble too.* (Reporting Data)

MS. POLLOCK: *What do you mean by other trouble, Daphne?* (Clarifying)

11. DAPHNE: *It will cause him some pain.* (Clarifying — Yes)

MS. POLLOCK: *Okay Daphne.* (Acknowledging) *You just reported a prediction about what might happen if he doesn't get some kind of treatment.* (Tuning In To Process)

12. DAPHNE: *Yeah.* (Clarifying — Yes. The student responded to the TIP as though it were Clarifying)

TEACHER: *Okay.*

13. CARLTON: *I think the first thing Gerry should do is check in with a clinic or see a doctor as soon as possible to take care of the*

	Student	Teacher

gonorrhea. (Reporting Course of Action)

14. FLOSSY: *You mean he shouldn't tell his girlfriend?* (Clarifying)

14. CL

15. CARLTON: *All I was saying was that he should get going on the treatment right away. He's right there in the doctor's office.* (Clarifying — Yes)

MS. POLLOCK; *Uh-huh. That's something he could do.* (Acknowledging)

15. CLY   A

16. JACK: *I think one thing for sure is he ought to tell any girl he's had contact with.* (Reporting Course of Action)

MS. POLLOCK: *Jack, would you be willing to share why you feel that way?* (Probe for Rationale)

16. RCA   PR

17. JACK: *Well, I think he has the responsibility to any girls he's had contact with to tell them. He might have given it to them or caught it from one of them and they might not know they have it. Anyway, he should let them know. That's what he should do and maybe he can help keep some other people from getting it.* (Probe for Rationale — Yes)

MS. POLLOCK: *Jack, let me try something and you help me understand if this is what you're saying. It seems to me that one of your values about people is that they behave responsibly toward others, especially where diseases are involved. Did I catch it?* (Inferring Values)

17. PRY   IV

18. JACK: *I never thought about it*

	Student	Teacher

that way. Yeah... I do think people should let others know about those kinds of things instead of being ashamed or something and not telling them. That's not right. (Inferring Values — Yes)

MS. POLLOCK: *Okay Jack.* (Acknowledging)

18. IVY — A

19. FERN: *A while ago somebody said that the doctor or clinic doesn't have to tell your parents if you have venereal disease. So, I think he should get the treatment, tell his girlfriend, or girlfriends, but not tell his parents.* (Reporting Course of Action)

MS. POLLOCK: *What do you think might happen, Fern, if he does what you said?* (Probe for Prediction)

19. RCA — PP

20. FERN: *He'd get better and his girlfriend would too if she gets treated and his father wouldn't be disappointed with him.* (Probe for Prediction — Yes)

MS. POLLOCK: *His mother and father wouldn't be disappointed?* (Clarifying)

20. PPY — CL

21. FERN: *Right, like most parents if they thought you had a venereal disease.* (Clarifying — Yes)

MS. POLLOCK: *Okay Fern.* (Acknowledging)

21. CLY — A

22. LEE: *I agree with Fern that he should take the treatment but not tell his parents* (Reporting Value Judgment) *because if he told his parents then they might not trust him or let him go out afterwards, or anything like that, because they*

	Student	Teacher

might be afraid that he'd do the same thing over again. So if he didn't tell his parents then he wouldn't be like grounded all the time for the rest of his life. (Reporting Prediction)

MS. POLLOCK: *Then you're agreeing with Jim?* (Clarifying)

23. LEE: *Yeah.* (Clarifying — Yes)

	Student	Teacher
22.	RVJ-RP	CL

MS. POLLOCK: *You're making a value judgment that that's a better approach as Fern said.* (Tuning in to Process) *Lee, can you think of any circumstances or conditions in which it would be a good idea to tell his parents?* (Probe for Conditions)

	Student	Teacher
23.	CLY	TIP-PC

24. LEE: *Yeah, if he were to have a lot of guilt by not telling his parents then I think he should tell them.* (Probe for Condition — Yes)

MS. POLLOCK: *All right.* (Acknowledging)

	Student	Teacher
24.	PCY	A

25. (To the whole group) *We're going to have to stop the discussion now. In the remaining time I'd like to invite you to respond to this question, "How do you feel about the discussion we just had?"* (Process Dialogue)

Structuring and Focus Setting for the Process Dialogue

Figure 17 shows this lesson recorded on an actual "T" System Lesson Analysis Record Form.

FIGURE 17

FS: *What should Gerald do?*

"T" System Lesson
Analysis Form

	Student	Teacher			Student	Teacher
1.		STR·O·FS	Jack	16.	RCA	PR
2.	GD	CL		17.	PRY	IV
3.	CLY	RDG		18.	IVY	A
4.	RCA	A	Fern	19.	RCA	PP
5.	RCA			20.	PPY	CL
6.	RVJ·RD·RP			21.	CLY	A
7.	RVJ·RD	A	Lee	22.	RVJ·RP	CL
8.	RP			23.	CLY	TIP·PC
9.	STRB	STR		24.	PCY	A
10.	RD	CL				
11.	CLY	A·TIP				
12.	CLY	A				
13.	RCA					
14.	CL					
15.	CLY	A				

STR–FS for Process Dialogue

Using the "T" System Lesson Analysis Record to Make Judgments About the Lesson

Once a "T" System Lesson Analysis Record has been developed, that data may be used to answer several questions about the values awareness lesson. Figure 18 is a list of these questions along with the identification of the data necessary to formulate a response to them. Depending on what the concerns of the teacher are at the time, the "T" System Lesson Analysis Record may be reviewed in terms of

FIGURE 18

Question	Data
Was the topic suitable for a values awareness lesson?	The frequent occurrence of RCA and RVJs in the student column indicates the degree to which students were using their values as they discussed the topic.
Was the lesson adequately structured?	The occurrence of a Structuring teaching behavior at the beginning of the lesson and the infrequent use of a Structuring teaching behavior to the entire class during the lesson indicates that the way the lesson was structured was appropriate for the students.
Was the proper climate created for the use of the Inferring Value teaching behavior?	The occasional occurrence of the IVN behavior in the student column indicates that the students felt comfortable in letting the teacher know when he or she was off course when an Inferring Value teaching behavior was used; that the proper climate has been effectively established. .
Did the teacher utilize the range of Values Awareness Goal Directed and Diagnostic teaching behaviors?	The occurrence of the range of teaching behaviors over the course of several lessons indicates that the teacher is working toward the range of goals suitable for values awareness lessons.
Were the Values Awareness Teaching Behaviors used appropriately?	The use of the teaching behaviors as outlined on the Values Awareness Teaching Behavior Interaction Patterns is one measure of the degree to which those teaching behaviors were used correctly.
Are the students able to discuss a controversial issue with each other in a responsible manner?	The infrequent occurrence of a Structuring teaching behavior directed to individual students to maintain or reinforce the lesson climate indicates the students are dealing with the topic and each other in a responsible manner.

one or more of these questions. This kind of a lesson record is not the only data base from which judgments about the degree of success of a lesson may be determined. It is one useful way, however, that some unique data about student and teaching behaviors may be recorded, organized and analyzed.

Other Ways to Make Judgments about Values Awareness Lessons

Two other ways to study a values awareness lesson center on the goals for instruction. Since there is a close relationship between the

Question	Data
Was the topic appropriate for the students?	The infrequent occurrence of (FS) or FS student behaviors indicates that the students understood the topic and were responding to it.
Are the students learning to recognize when they or others in the group make a shift from the discussion topic?	The occurrence of the FS student behavior indicates that the students are becoming sensitive to any shift they or others make in the discussion topic.
Were the Probe, Clarifying, and Inferring Value teaching behaviors used effectively?	The frequent occurrence of "Y" behaviors and infrequent occurrence of "N" or "S" behaviors in the student column indicates that the probe, Clarifying, and Inferring Value teaching behaviors were formulated and used effectively.
Are the students beginning to explicate their own values or the values of others during or after the lessons?	The occurrence of the Reporting Value student behavior indicates that the students are developing a concept of value that they can use to gain new insight into themselves and others.
Was the teacher able to limit his or her behavior mainly to the use of the Values Awareness Teaching Behaviors?	The infrequent occurrence of the "O" and absence of ϕ (behaviors inconsistent with values awareness lessons) in the teacher column indicates that the teacher has been effective in confining his or her behavior to those behaviors appropriate for a values awareness lesson.
Are the students learning to communicate with each other and with the teacher more effectively?	A decrease in the occurrence of the Clarifying behavior either by the teacher or the students as compared to earlier lessons indicates that the students are becoming more effective in communicating their ideas.

FIGURE 19

TEACHING BEHAVIOR/GOALS CHECKLIST

Tally each Occurrence	Teaching Behavior	Goal
_____	Tunning In To Process	• Helping the students become aware of the processes they or others use during a discussion.
_____	Probe for Rationale and Inferring Value	• Helping the students recognize that the decisions they make are based in part on the values they hold.
		• Helping the students become aware of some of the values they hold.
		• Developing the students' ability to more systematically explicate their own values and infer the values of others.
_____	Probe for Prediction	• Developing the students ability to weigh possible/probable consequences before implementing a course of action.
_____	Probe for Data	• Helping the students become aware of the role of data in decision making.
_____	Probe for Data Source	• Developing the students' ability to analyze the source of data as one way of judging the validity of that data.
_____	Probe for Conditions	• Developing the students' ability to explicate the conditions that affect (1) the successful implementation of a course of action or (2) the prioritization of one's values.
		• Sensitizing the students to the role of conditions in decision making.
_____	Focus Setting	• Developing the students' ability to recognize when they or others are shifting the topic of the discussion.
_____	Probe for Values	• Helping the students recognize that the decisions they make are based in part on the values they hold.
		• Developing the students' ability to more systematically explicate their own values and the values of others.

teaching behaviors and the lesson goals, another way to make a judgment about a lesson is to prepare a checklist of the teaching behaviors. A tally mark by one of those teaching behaviors on the list become a record of each time the teacher has directed his or her actions toward one or more of the goals for values awareness.

Figure 19 is a checklist of the critical Values Awareness Teaching Behaviors. The comments in the right margin indicate the goal served when each of the specific teaching behaviors are utilized.

Another kind of checklist can be developed from a list of goals for values awareness lessons. In this case, however, the attention of the observer is directed only to what the students say or do that may be interpreted as evidence of their progress toward the goals of the teaching strategy. A tally is made by the appropriate goal when any such behavior occurs. Figure 20 is an illustrative goals checklist.

FIGURE 20

STUDENT BEHAVIOR/GOALS CHECKLIST

_____	● Awareness that the decisions they make are based in part on the values they hold.
_____	● Awareness of the role of data in decision making.
_____	● Awareness of the processes they or others use during a discussion and the effects of those processes on others.
_____	● Awareness of some of the values they hold.
_____	● Ability to systematically explicate their own values.
_____	● Ability to systematically infer the values of others.
_____	● Ability to analyze the source of data as one way of judging the validity of that data.
_____	● Ability to weigh possible/probable consequences before implementing a course of action.
_____	● Ability to recognize when they or others in a discussion are shifting topics.
_____	● Ability to use language patterns that enable them to disagree with others while maintaining open lines of communication.
_____	● Ability to interact effectively with others who's values differ.
_____	● Ability to communicate their feelings, opinions and attitudes effectively.
_____	● Ability to explicate the conditions that affect (1) the successful implementation of a course of action or (2) the prioritization of one's values.
_____	● Awareness of the role of conditions in decision making.

While it is obvious that the Student Behavior/Goals Checklist is used to record student's goal-related behavior during the discussion portion of a values awareness lesson, this checklist can also be used during The Process Dialogue. However, in addition to gleaning evidence of the aforementioned goals, the students may give evidence of the affective effect of the teaching strategy during the Process Dialogue as they make comments about how they felt about the lesson.

Finally, a way to judge one of the effects of the Values Awareness Teaching Strategy over the course of a semester or school year is to direct attention to changes in the students' level of values development. (See "A Notion of Natural Values Development.") To do so it is necessary to analyze the rationale students report for a course of action they recommend or a value judgment they make or support. The following guidelines are used to conduct this analysis. Anytime a

FIGURE 21

GUIDELINES FOR
DISCRIMINATING THE LEVEL OF VALUES DEVELOPMENT

Level	Level Indicator
I. Developing Behavior Patterns: Pre-Values	Cites pleasure/pain, approval or disapproval as a rationale for a course of action or value judgment: ● Because it hurts/feels good. ● Because my Mother/Father says I should/shouldn't.
II. Developing Behavior Standards: Intuitive Values	Cites a rule or norm as rationale for a course of action or value judgment: ● Because all the kids eat them. ● Well, it's a good rule to brush your teeth after eating.
III. Developing Insight into Behavior Standards: Awareness Values	Cites an important characteristic as a rationale for a course of action or value judgment: ● Because it will protect you from getting infected. ● Because she is an independent thinker.
IV. Developing a Consistency Between Behavior and Values: Functional Values	Cites a value as a rationale for a course of action or value judgment: ● Because one of my values about health measures is that they provide you as well as others protection against illness. ● Because one of my values about physicians is that they are dependable.

student reports a rationale either voluntarily or in response to a Probe for Rationale teaching behavior, his or her rationale is tallied in terms of the four levels outlined (Figure 21).

This last technique is perhaps the easiest to use and offers the teacher very significant data about his or her students. Used at the beginning and end of the semester, evidence of the students' level of values development can be assessed. This, therefore, becomes yet another way the effectiveness of the Values Awareness Teaching Strategy may be judged.

Each way of working to evaluate a lesson yields a slightly different view of that lesson. Each produces a different statement about what went on. It makes sense, therefore, for a teacher to use a variety of techniques to generate feedback about the lesson, including other approaches not described here. To do so produces a more holistic picture of the impact of the Values Awareness Teaching Strategy on children and youth.

References

1. Means RK: Historical Perspectives on School Health. New Jersey: Charles B. Slack, Inc., 1975, pp 1-3.
2. Goodlad JI: School Curriculum Reform in the United States. New York: The Fund for the Advancement of Education, 1964, pp 24, 26, 27.
3. Joint Committee on Health Education Terminology Definitions. Health Education Monographs. San Francisco: Society for Public Health Education, Inc. No. 33, 1973.
4. Committee to Develop a Statement of Philosophy for Health Education. Philosophical Perspectives. Health Education, 6:12-14, January/February, 1975.
5. Russell RD: Health Education. Washington, D.C.: Joint Committee on Health Problems in Education of the National Education Association and the American Medical Association, 1975.
6. School Health Section, American Public Health Association. Position Paper: Education for Health in the School Community Setting. Washington, D.C.: American Public Health Association, 1974.
7. Sliepcevich EM: Health Education, A Conceptual Approach to Curriculum Design. St. Paul, Minnesota: 3-M Press, 1967, p 84.
8. School Health Education Study, Health Education: A Conceptual Approach To Curriculum Design. St. Paul: 3M Education Press, 1967.
9. Simon, Howe, Kirschenbaum: Values Clarification, A Handbook of Strategies for Teachers. New York: Hart Publishing Co., 1972.
10. Pfeiffer and Jones: A Handbook of Structured Experiences for Human Relations Training, Vol. I, Vol. II, Vol. III, Vol. IV. LaJolla, California: University Associates, 1974.